GET FIT
GET HEALTHY
GET HAPPY

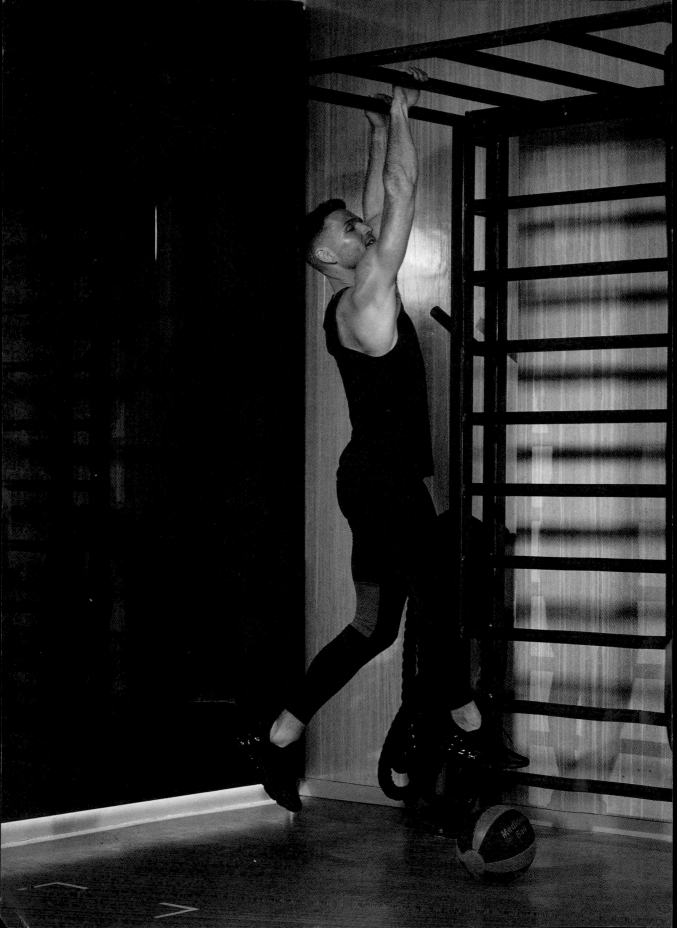

The ultimate guide to being in the best shape of your life

GET FIT
GET HEALTHY
GET HAPPY

TRAIN WRIGHT WITH
MARK WRIGHT

Thorsons

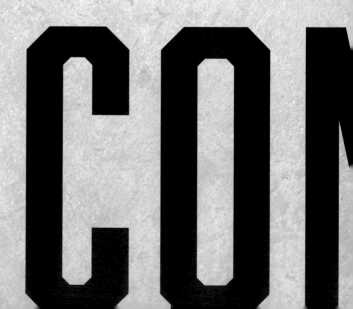

TRAIN WRIGHT

TENTS

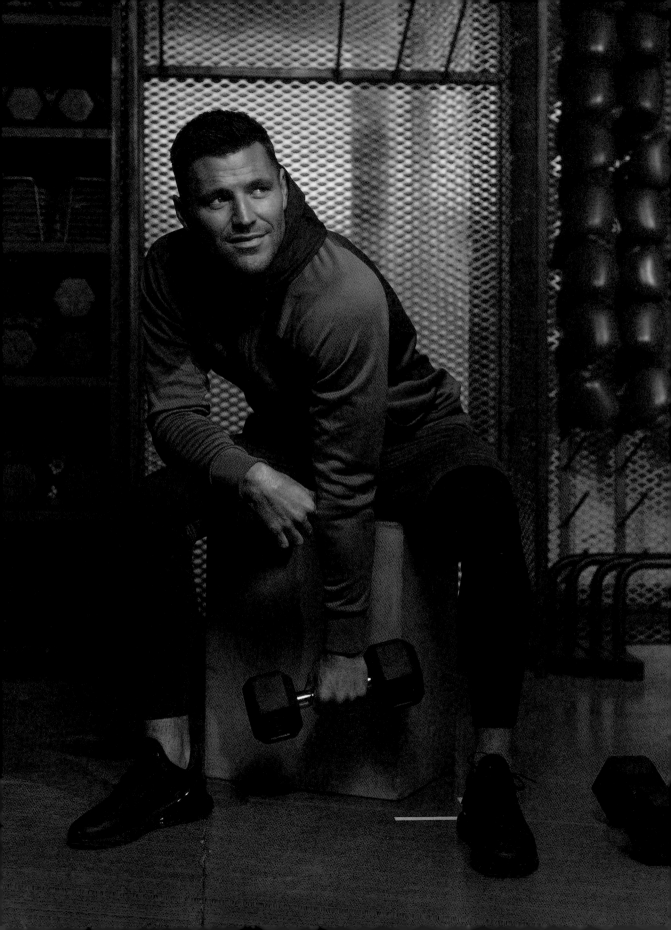

INTRODUCTION

Hi.

Firstly, I want to say well done! You've picked up this book, you've taken it home and you have opened it up to read the first chapter. This is the first and most important step towards leading a healthier lifestyle and I'm so glad it was my book that you decided to buy because I guarantee that by the end of it you are going to be in the best shape of your life, both physically and mentally. And the good news is, while it really will change your life, you won't have to make any drastic lifestyle overhauls and you'll still be able to enjoy the things you love. That's the beauty of the Train Wright lifestyle and it is why I can't wait to share it with you.

One thing that I hear a LOT from people who don't know me is this: 'I bet he spends his life in the gym, never goes out and lives on salads.' I have to laugh because the reality is that nothing could be further from the truth. I generally work out about four or five times a week, but it's usually from home and for just 30 minutes each time. (I've recently returned to playing professional football, so my training levels have increased.) I love cooking and eating healthy food, but I can't remember the last time I had a salad and most of all, I NEVER sacrifice my social life. I love ordering a takeaway with Michelle (my wife) on a Saturday night and watching Netflix, or having a pizza and beers with my mates while watching footy at the weekend. That's what life is all about and any diet or fitness plan that tells you to give these things up is only setting you up to fail. Obviously I don't eat like this every day, but I make sure I practice balance, and that is what this book and the Train Wright Six-week Plan is going to teach you.

> Of course, I've made all the classic mistakes along the way. Depriving yourself of the things you love doesn't work (believe me, I've tried).

I'm not going to pretend I've always known how to live a well-balanced life, and nowhere in this book will you find me claiming to be the world's best personal trainer or chef, but what I hope the next few pages will give you is an understanding of how my life, from my upbringing to my career as a footballer and my life in the public eye, has taught me more about health, fitness and diet than most. It's been a hell of a journey but one that – I believe – can help you to make small changes that will lead to you achieving huge benefits to your life.

Of course, I've made all the classic mistakes along the way. Depriving yourself of the things you love doesn't work (believe me, I've tried); thinking you can eat and drink what you want and not see it impact your figure doesn't work (believe me, I've experienced it); believing that spending money on expensive gym memberships and diet products will give you results will only leave you disappointed (believe me, I've learnt this too). But I've always made it my mission in life to learn from my mistakes, and that's what's led me to developing the Train Wright way of life and why I know it's the best way to achieve long-term goals. I've made the mistakes so you no longer have to.

This book isn't going to teach you how to give things up, it's going to teach you how to go and get them – and then some. I cannot wait for you to join me because I know how amazing you are going to feel as soon as you get started.

Let's do this.

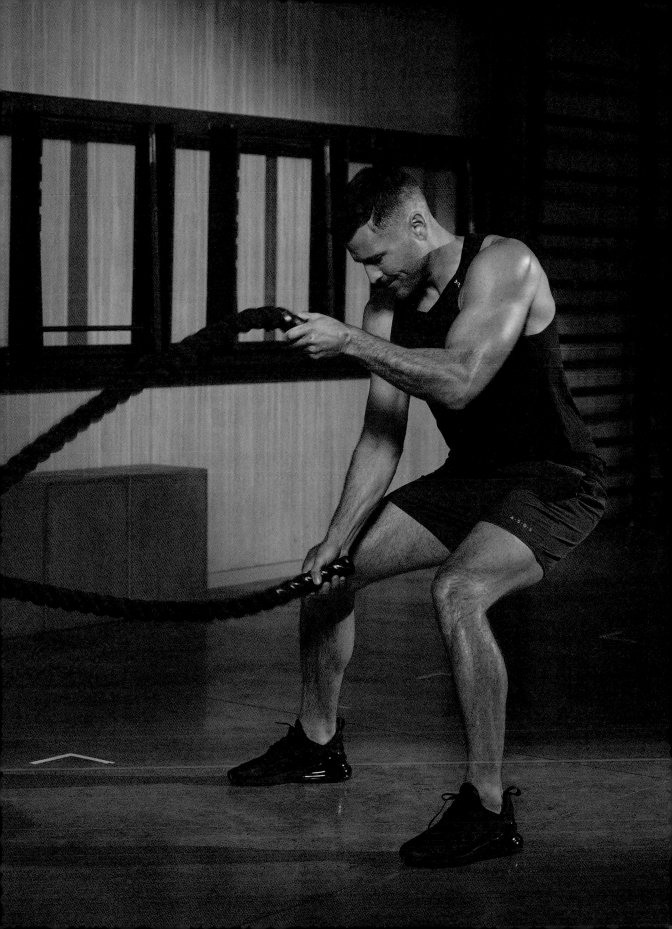

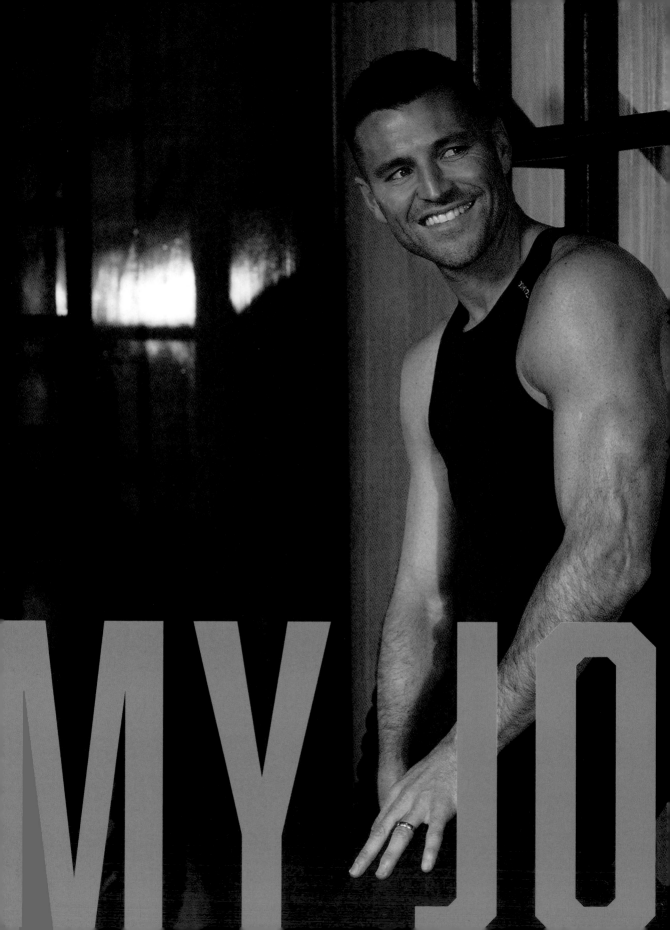

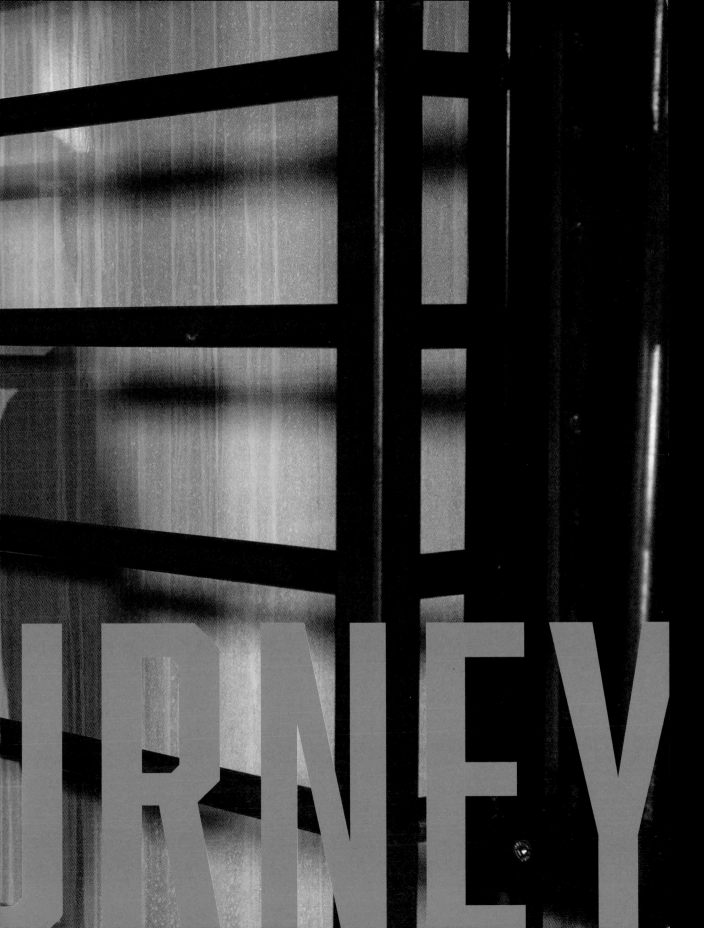

CHAPTER 1 – FROM WRONG LIFE TO WRIGHT LIFE

I knew I couldn't write a book about finding motivation to live and exercise healthily without sharing my personal story. So much of the way we live our lives is based on the journey we've gone on to get where we are now.

It's so easy for us to go through life without thinking back to each individual experience and how it has shaped us. I noticed that when people ask me about my personality I'd often respond with, 'I've always been competitive', or 'I've always been a driven person', but that's just not true. No one is born competitive or driven. It's only since setting up Train Wright and questioning where my motivation and competitiveness comes from that I've realised so much of it is based on my experiences in the early years of my life.

It might surprise a lot of people, but I'm usually quite private about how I grew up. It didn't feel right, however, not to share my backstory with you when, later in the book, I'm going to be asking you to think about yours.

There are two experiences in my life that make me as driven as I am and I'm going to tell you exactly what they are and how they've helped me find a healthy, balanced lifestyle.

THE EARLY YEARS

I was very lucky and grew up in a family I could only have dreamed of being born into.

I came into the world in January 1987, the second child of my mum Carol and dad Mark. My sister Jessica is 18 months older than me, my brother, Josh, came along two years after me and my sister Natalya, 20, is the youngest. Family was, and still is, absolutely everything to me.

As well as being super close to my immediate family, I have a huge wider family. My dad has three brothers, which means I have a lot of cousins, and we all grew up together as we lived around the corner from each other. There were so many of us on family holidays that we used to call ourselves 'The Hillbillies' when we travelled abroad.

My dad and two of his brothers were all, at some point in their lives, professional sportsmen, and one of my uncles was a pro golfer. This meant that, from an early age, I was surrounded by sport and – much more significantly – competition.

A competitive attitude was bred into me from the beginning, and while it has helped me achieve so much in my life and career, I do admit that one of my negative traits is often being too competitive. We recently went on a huge family holiday abroad and the whole trip revolved around sports. Swimming races, kayaking, football games,

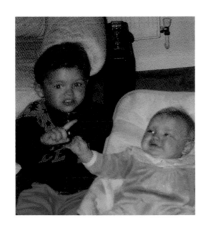

tennis tournaments, golf matches – you name it, we did it, and every single member of my family was in it to win it. It never gets nasty, and it's always fun, but absolutely no one wants to lose. On the flight home my wife Michelle and my sister's fiancé said they were going to have to take lessons in all the different sports before the next holiday so they could up their game.

It's just part of how we bond, and I love it.

I had a fantastic upbringing. My parents were very supportive of my siblings and me when we were kids, spending their evenings and weekends driving me round to every different club and class you can imagine.

I did cricket, boxing, football, tennis, rugby, athletics – even ballet. There wasn't anything I didn't want to try.

I always gave my everything as I wanted to be the best player in class. Unfortunately that determination didn't extend to my schoolwork. I always got on with my teachers – I remember at parent's evenings they'd always say, 'He's very cheeky', and 'He's certainly the entertainer of the classroom' – but I just didn't love academia. It didn't suit me. I'll hold my hands up, I was a mischievous, cheeky young lad, but I never stood for bullying.

I was taught by my granddad that you should stand up to bullies and never walk by when someone is being picked on. When I was 10 I walked into the PE changing room at school and saw two kids physically bullying another boy and I completely lost my temper. I ended up punching one of the bullies and was landed with a week's suspension. I had to tell my parents what happened but luckily, when my dad sat me down, he said: 'I don't want to tell you what you did was right, but you did the right thing by standing up to bullies.' I'd never encourage physical retaliation now, but I couldn't stand by and watch bullying.

My family history is rooted in the East End of London. When I went on the TV show *Who Do You Think You Are?*, I found out that, way back, my family came from Spanish descent, but in much more recent years they were market traders. This made so much sense to me as my dad was

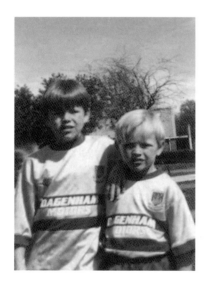

brought up as a hard grafter and he has always been incredibly driven to work for himself.

Up until the age of five, I had everything. My dad owned his own business he had built from scratch and did really well for himself. We lived in a detached five-bed house in Essex with a swimming pool and I never went without. I even had one of those big electric cars for kids from Toys R Us. When I was six we suddenly moved out of the family home and into a rented house down the road. I remember wondering why we were moving, but Mum and Dad never let on that anything was wrong. The following year we moved out again, this time into a two-bedroom apartment. There were five of us at this point, so all three kids had to share a bedroom and I was very aware by this point that something wasn't right. Just a few months later, we didn't have a home. It feels weird to say we were homeless, because it never felt that way, but technically we were. My brother Josh and I moved into my nanny Pat and granddad Charlie's house with my mum, while my sister Jess moved in with my dad and his parents, Eddie and Irene.

Mum and Dad never sat us down and said anything, but almost overnight we had lost everything. I was on a blow-up bed with my brother in the spare room and my mum was on a single bed in my nan and granddad's room in their two-bed house. I saw the pain my mum suffered in those years and it has never left me. I vividly remember an argument when I was about seven. My granddad Charlie came downstairs and there was a wet shower towel on the floor. He picked it up and said to my mum, 'For God's sake, another towel in the middle of the floor'. He was having a dig at me and my brother for being messy. Mum just broke down crying and said, 'What do you want me to do? I have nowhere else for us to go.'

I strongly remember how I felt an immediate vulnerability but equally felt a need to be strong, at the same time.

I took on a man-of-the-house role, made sure the family stayed strong, and grew up very quickly. I later found out that – due to the recession – they lost it all. I saw it take everything from my family. We lived without a family home, in separate houses, for two years and I will always remember thinking, the only reason we weren't literally homeless was because of the amazing family support system we had around us.

This experience did two things to me. Firstly, it made me incredibly driven when it comes to work. I understood that hard work is necessary to get you where you want to go and I learnt how quickly it can be taken away from you. Over my career I have been so grateful for every single job I have been offered that I don't know when to say no. I have often taken on too much and have had to rein it in, but that early experience in life gave me this determined mentality to always work hard and never take any job for granted. Secondly, it taught me that family is everything. I learnt the hard way that, no matter what happened, my family would be there for me and that has been something I have made sure I've always carried with me.

My mum and dad are the most in-love couple I have ever seen. Their relationship has always been an inspiration to me and looking back now I can't begin to imagine how hard it must have been for them losing everything and living apart with three kids. Yet they still stayed so in love and never let the situation come between their love for each other.

STARTING A CAREER

Watching my family lose everything was one of the toughest things I'd ever been through.

I remember a kid called Hugh coming up to me in the playground and saying, 'I've heard your mum and dad have gone bankrupt,' and that was heartbreaking for me, but watching my dad refuse to give up, pick himself up and start from scratch, trying every avenue he could to make money, was a complete inspiration.

At the age of 12 I started washing cars. Every Tuesday and Friday I got dropped off in the local rich area and I'd knock on every door asking if people wanted their cars washing. I'd wash five or six cars a night and one guy even got me cutting his lawn too. By 13 I'd saved up £700 and I bought my first car, a second-hand Peugeot 206 that I knew was cheap. I couldn't drive, but I knew I could make a profit. I sold it on Auto Trader a week later for £950. I started car dealing after this and made myself £6,000 in two and a half years, and by the age of 16 I was able to buy myself a Ford Fiesta Zetec. I had this unstoppable force within me to succeed and that has translated into every aspect of my life.

FOOTBALL

Alongside this story runs my journey with professional football.

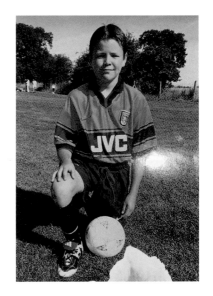

My first word was 'ball' and I was completely obsessed with the game from a very early age. Every picture of me as a kid has a football in it, and I've even still got my first ever football boots from when I was two. Of course I was way too small to be able to wear them, but that's how much I loved it.

I was scouted for West Ham United at the age of seven and played for them until, at the age of 10, I went to Arsenal. At 14 I moved to Charlton Athletic. At the time, Arsenal was one of the biggest clubs in the country; they were in their glory days with Thierry Henry, and a lot of people questioned my decision, but this was the time when, financially, my family were really struggling. My dad desperately wanted to keep me at private school but his money had run out, so when Charlton offered to pay for mine and my brother's school fees, it was a no-brainer for my parents. I had an amazing two years there, until I left school at 16 and that's when I moved to Tottenham FC. Here I had the season of my life: I was captain of the team, one of the highest-performing players on the squad and I was all set to become the next left back of Tottenham. That's when the second shock of my life happened.

Alongside this story runs my journey with professional football. My first word was 'ball' and I was completely obsessed with the game from a very early age.

After an incredible season I agreed to go away to the Costa Blanca in Spain for a month in the summer with my cousin Elliot and mate Jack. I'd worked incredibly hard, and during every other off season I'd always kept myself in shape, but this summer, because I was at the top of the team in terms of performance, I thought, 'I deserve a break.' It was one of the biggest mistakes of my life. At this point I'd never drunk alcohol, and I'd always eaten a healthy diet and taken care of myself. That summer I drank alcohol every day, partied nearly every night and ate a diet of burgers, chips and chicken nuggets around the pool. When I went back for the first day of training after summer I'd put on a stone and a half in weight, felt horrendous and my fitness levels were shocking. In our cardio drills the goalkeepers were outrunning me and I knew I was in serious trouble. The manager took me to one side as he was so shocked, and told me I had to turn up an hour earlier to join the 'fat boys club' to do extra training and burn off the fat. But mentally, I just couldn't pull it back. I'd ignore their nutritional advice and pick up a cheese and onion pasty on my way in. When the physio and manager weren't looking I'd stop cycling on the bike and when I got a shin splint injury a month later I just used it as an excuse to avoid the fitness drills. The team were shocked and a few months later I ended up moving to Southend United. That was a big blow for me because I was no longer at a premier league club. I realised I'd thrown it all away and because I had lost myself physically, I mentally gave up too. I ended up dropping down the leagues and losing my love for it.

My football earnings were no longer enough to sustain me, so I tried to find other avenues to earn a living. That's when I found nightclub promoting in Essex. I earnt more money doing that than low-level football, so I ended up dropping further down the leagues and being semi-pro. This is where my workaholic side really came out in force. I trained Tuesday and Thursday nights for football, worked the nightclubs on Friday and Saturday nights, but realised I wasn't doing anything to earn money during the day. I got a nine-to-five job as a stockbroker from Monday to Friday in the City and completely ran myself into the ground. On a Thursday I'd get a train in at 7am, finish at 6pm and get back on a train to Essex. I'd run from the station to the ground in my suit, quickly change and then train till 9:30pm. I'd then jump back on a train to London to go to the nightclub I promoted and work till 3am. Then I'd do it all again the next day. I didn't want to turn any work down as I had a constant anxiety about losing it all and having no money. I did this, working three jobs, for eight months, until I burned out. Mentally, I wanted to do it, but physically I couldn't keep it up without sleep or a healthy diet. I quit the stockbroking job and focused on club promoting and football while I figured out what I was going to do next. And then my life changed all over again.

THE TOWIE YEARS

I was 19 and renting a two-bed flat with my mate Tony in Harlow, Essex. After my football career had failed, I was throwing all my efforts into club promoting and working on getting fitter and having a healthier work/life balance.

At the time, reality TV was just taking off in the US. I got into a conversation one night with a guy at one of my nightclubs who worked in TV. We talked about how good it could be to do an Essex version and this got my mind racing with ideas. He set up meetings with some of his producers and they decided to film a pilot episode.

I watched the first episode of *TOWIE* when it launched and thought it was a bit of fun, then went to bed. The next day I woke up and my Twitter had gone crazy. I had thousands of followers out of nowhere and when I walked down my local high street in Essex, people were stopping me for pictures. I couldn't believe how big it had gone. I remember texting my mum that night after walking into a nightclub and realising everyone was staring at me; I said: 'Mum, WTF, I think I'm famous.' Within a few months I was being booked for nightclub appearances instead of being the one booking them, and everything just went crazy. If I'm honest, it gave me real anxiety at the start because I didn't know what to do with all the attention.

After the first series ended I was invited to an ITV party. I remember turning up, looking around the room and seeing huge names like Piers Morgan, Holly Willoughby, Phillip Schofield and Dermot O'Leary and thinking, 'I'm just a guy who has been on *TOWIE*, these guys have made serious careers out of TV and I'm in a room with them.' For the whole journey home from that event all that was going around in my head was, 'I have been given a platform here and I have two choices. I either let it play out and wait for nightclub appearances to come to me, or I go out and make something much bigger from it.' That night I realised I was mentally and physically ready to give everything to this opportunity and was determined not to let it slip away.

> I realised pretty early on that, if I wanted to make a career for myself outside of *TOWIE*, I would need to prove myself.

HEADING TO THE JUNGLE

After series two of *TOWIE* aired in 2011, the show won the Audience Award at the BAFTAs. It was the first structured reality TV show in the UK and it was a really exciting time. I loved being part of the show and I know how lucky I was to have been on it, but let me tell you, trying to be taken seriously as a presenter after being 'Mark Wright from *TOWIE*' was not easy. There was a lot of stigma attached to the show and the press loved playing on the 'young, pretty and stupid' stereotype that was associated with the Essex crowd. I realised pretty early on that, if I wanted to make a career for myself outside of TOWIE, I would need to prove myself. I agreed to do a final series of the show, and once filming was over I signed up to go on *I'm A Celebrity... Get Me Out Of Here!* It wasn't a quick decision, I debated long and hard whether to do it or not, but I really wanted to be able to show the real me, aside from the character I had to play up to on *TOWIE*.

I knew it was a risk, but I really wanted the opportunity to take on a new challenge and put myself out there for people to see me as me. I told myself, 'If people don't like me, I can take that because I know that I'll be completely myself, and if they do like me, then I'll know I stand a chance of really making something of myself, because it won't be *TOWIE* Mark that everyone is expecting any more, it will be me.'

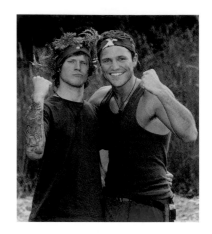

What I wasn't ready for was how difficult the Jungle was going to be. It is so much harder than anyone can imagine. The boredom is really tough. But much, much harder than that was the hunger. We were all way hungrier than you can portray on TV and that was another whole new feeling to me. When I talk to people about getting fitter and healthier, I always preach that you should never go hungry. A healthy diet for me is not about starving myself or limiting anything because I know the importance of fuelling your body. So dealing with extreme hunger, with nothing to take my mind off it, pushed me to somewhere I'd not been before. I felt stressed and my mood was so low that I went to the producers midway through and told them: 'I don't think I can do this.' Each time I came close to quitting I kept thinking, 'If I quit on this, I could be quitting a huge opportunity and I can't be the man I was when I mucked up my football career.' I spent hours during the days of boredom thinking about my dad and how he had worked so hard but lost everything, but he had never given up, he never quit, he always kept fighting. It was a mental strength I had to find and, having these experiences in my past, they were what helped me dig deep and not quit. And I am beyond grateful that I did. I was the runner-up on the show and when I came out I was immediately offered three TV shows. It wasn't just an experience that helped me show people who I really was, it was an experience that taught ME who I was, what I was capable of mentally and how valuable my past was in shaping my future.

> **It was an experience that taught ME who I was, what I was capable of mentally and how valuable my past was in shaping my future.**

TAKING THE MIC

I'm not going to pretend that my career path has been as easy as one stint in the Jungle.

Yes, it was a huge stepping stone out of *TOWIE*, but I now had a whole new learning curve coming my way. As I said, I was offered jobs immediately after the Jungle: presenter on *Take Me Out: The Gossip*, presenter of a new game show, and my own show, *Mark's Hollywood Nights*. I was so grateful, I couldn't wait to get started and, typically, I said yes to all of them, even though it meant crazy schedules and barely any time off. I didn't once stop to think, 'I've been offered all this work, but I've never presented a TV show in my life.' I knew I was going to work harder than ever and give it everything I possibly could, but that didn't stop it from being really bloody hard. Presenting is not a walk in the park and it takes a lot of experience to get anywhere near good enough to get your own show. And here I was with three of them.

The first show I filmed was a game show and I'll admit right now that I was nowhere near ready. I just wasn't experienced enough or good enough and, thank goodness, it never made it to air on TV. *Hollywood Nights* was filmed with me and my mates on holiday in LA and when I got back I started filming *Take Me Out: The Gossip*. I still wasn't good enough in front of the camera but luckily, *Take Me Out* was such a big show that the content just about carried my spin-off through. Unfortunately I couldn't say the same for *Hollywood Nights*. I remember reading the headlines the day after it aired saying, 'Is this the worst show on TV?' It felt like everything was crashing down around me and when someone in the industry tried to make me feel better by saying, 'Don't worry, mate, everyone has a failed TV show on the way up,' I had to reply saying, 'Yeah, but I've had three in a row.' This is where my determination kicked in again. I took every single bit of negative feedback on board and signed up for a long course of presenting lessons. I continued with my Heart FM radio show, but everything else was put to one side so I could focus on learning the craft. I took it ridiculously seriously and made sure I was doing workouts every morning to kickstart my day, eating well to give me energy and sleeping well to keep me focused. So when, four years later in 2017, I got a call offering me the job on new primetime TV show called *Cannonball*, this time I felt ready. They said it was a Saturday night show on ITV and I was perfect for it. I was pumped. I prepared for six months for the show then, while I was standing in the gym car park with my wife Michelle, I got a call from the big boss of ITV. He said, 'Mark, take this as a bit of a bummer, but we're giving the show to Freddie Flintoff… But take it as a positive that we know you are ready.' I couldn't believe it. I knew opportunities like this didn't come around often. This time though, I wasn't going to give up like I did when I gave up on football, at the first sign of failure. I needed to go back to the drawing board and work out how I could show people how serious I was about this. And that's when the American chapter of my life began.

THE AMERICAN DREAM

I'd always wanted to work in America. To me it was exciting, it was different and it was a way to prove to UK TV stations that I was capable of taking on big jobs. I talked to Michelle about it and she said, 'Mark, go.' I confided in her that I didn't know anyone there and I was worried about not making it, but she just looked at me and said, 'You will.' The next day I called my agent and said, 'I'm quitting my radio show and all my other commitments and I'm going to America.' They told me not to go, that if I went there I'd fail, then have to come back, but I was determined to show everyone that I could do it. The next day I was on a flight to LA.

I called an agent on my way to the airport and told him I was coming to America. I'd just quit three jobs and I needed to get a job. It sounds crazy when I tell it back, but the reason I quit it all was because I knew this wasn't going to be easy. I didn't want to have the safe option of coming home back to my jobs, so I eliminated that opportunity. I wanted it to be 'do or die' so I threw myself in at the deep end. I had a lot of meetings to start with, but I remember a huge turning point was a day at Universal Studios. By chance I stumbled across a crew who were filming the spin-off show for *Extra*. Mario Lopez was the host at the time and as I watched him I said to myself, 'That's the job I want.' I told my agent, who managed to get me a meeting with the female boss of the network and I still remember the day I walked in and told her who I was. I told her I'd dropped everything to come to America and work and that I was prepared to do anything, and work harder than anyone else, if I was given this opportunity. She agreed to give me a shot and told me to get some celebrity interviews for the channel. That's when she set the bar high. She said, 'I'm gonna give you a chance. You've got one week to get a star we'd play on our show. Produce it. Direct it. And interview them.' She told me she wanted James Corden, David Beckham or Adele. I knew she was giving me a huge challenge to see if I was up to it, so I exhausted all my contacts and spent all day and night calling everyone I could until Niall Horan from One Direction agreed to let me film on the set of his new music video and have the first interview.

When you want something that is within your reach, if you work hard and you put your mind to it and you fight for it, you CAN get it.

She loved it, but said the network didn't have any spaces for presenters and if anything came up, they'd let me know.

I had to be up early the next morning to fly back to London. I remember I was on the plane, the seatbelt was fastened, but we hadn't started to taxi when my phone rang. It was her assistant and she said, 'Mark, where are you?' I told her I was on the flight home and she said, 'Oh that's a shame, don't worry.' I was like: 'No, no. What were you going to say?' And that's when she told me that they had a one-off job interviewing James Corden. I told her I'd take it, I got up, grabbed my stuff, got off the plane and raced out of the airport. I gave that interview everything and they loved it, but yet again, they told me they had no permanent jobs. Four weeks went by and nothing. I flew home for a few days to see Michelle, and that's when I heard the news that one of the female presenters on *Extra* had been fired and they needed a replacement. I packed a bag immediately, drove to the airport and tried to get the next flight to LA. I tried every airline, but no one could fit me on. Instead of going home, I slept on those awful plastic airport seats until finally, early the next morning, a flight had a spare seat. I went straight from LA airport to the network boss's office and she looked shocked to see me. I told her I couldn't just sit at home knowing this job was available, and she told me to tell her, right there, how much I wanted it.

I felt like all the experience of my childhood, seeing my dad lose everything, letting my football career go down the drain, failing my first presenter job, all of that had led to this moment and I just poured my heart out to her. She didn't say anything at first but then she said, 'You've got it. Now get out of my office before I change my mind.' I left, called Michelle and burst into tears. I'd done it. For me, in that moment, I knew that when you want something badly enough – and I'm not talking about winning the lottery or getting a number-one single – but when you want something that is within your reach, if you work hard and you put your mind to it and you fight for it, you CAN get it.

SHARING MY FITNESS JOURNEY

I've always kept fit. Throughout my entire career, after that one summer in Spain where I threw it all away by letting fitness fall by the wayside, I have made sure exercise is scheduled into my life.

I put it in my diary, and while it might mean I only fit in a 20-minute workout in the morning on really busy days, I make sure I get it done. I believe this has been a huge driving force behind my success because it has kept my confidence up, has supported my drive and passion to work hard and has kept me focused. From the *TOWIE* days, all the way through to now, I've had messages from fans and friends asking for advice on keeping fit and healthy. It is such a passion that I've always tried to reply to as many of them as possible.

Then 2020 happened and everything changed. A huge chunk of my workload was taken away and suddenly I had all this free time. As you know, I'm not someone who gets a kick out of sitting still, so from day one I knew this was my chance to help people stuck in lockdown needing advice on how to stay healthy. I told my Instagram followers that I would be hosting live streams of my daily workouts that they could follow along for free. I honestly thought a few people would do them and it would keep me busy for a few weeks, but thousands of people joined me every day and the messages I received, telling me that I was helping them stay physically and mentally strong, were amazing. I kept up the workouts throughout the whole of lockdown; I even invited my celebrity friends and other trainers on and it formed this community of people all over the world joining in. I had 60-year-old women in Australia joining in, new mums and their kids, and everyone in between. I had to keep going,

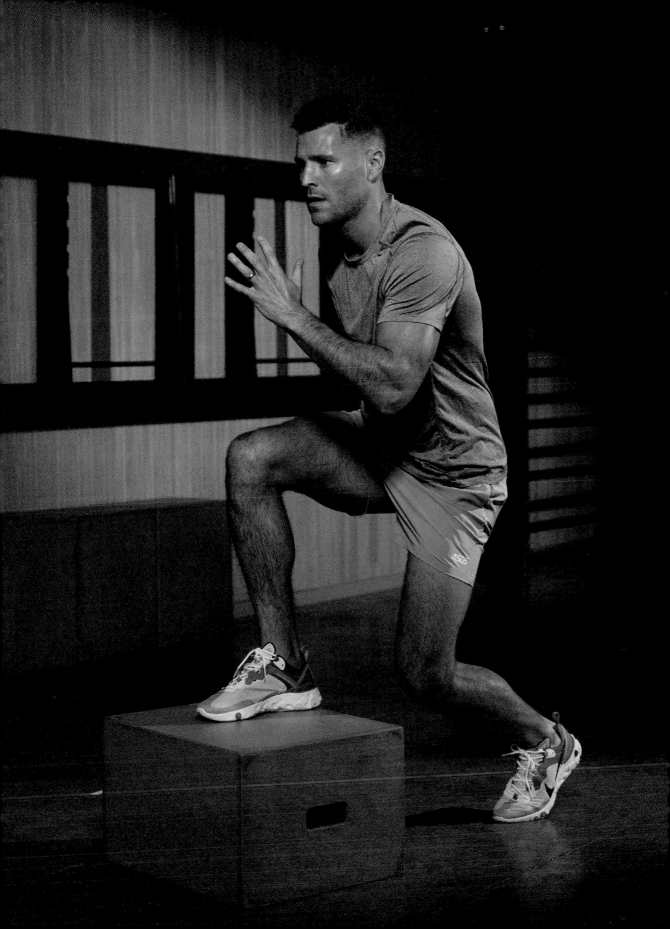

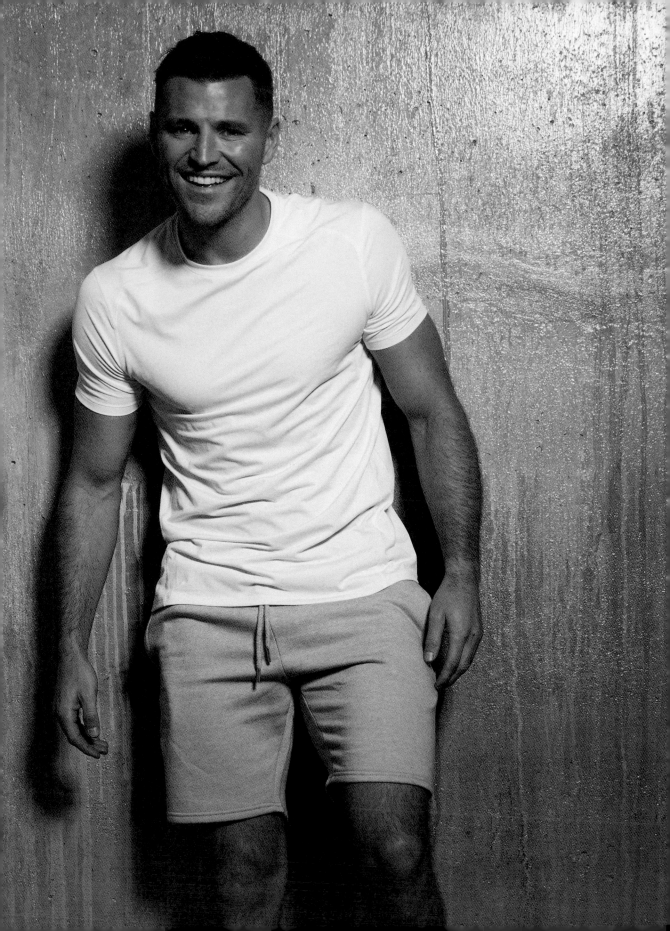

and that's what motivated me to set up my online fitness platform, Train Wright. I'm still overwhelmed by how many people have signed up, and every time I get messages from people telling me how much weight they've lost or how much it's changed their lives, I get such a buzz because I know how powerful that feeling is.

It's been over 11 years since I fully retired from serious football and not a day's gone by when I don't miss it. The fact that I never played a professional game in the league has always niggled at me. More recently, my internal competitive voice was stronger than ever, saying, 'If you don't do it now, you never will.' So, at the age of 33, I knew it had to be now. In October 2020, I got the opportunity to train with Crawley Town FC. I couldn't wait to get onto the pitch, but at first it was just for fitness training and because I knew it would help scratch the itch I was feeling from missing the game. I put everything and more into the training, both with the team and by myself, and I made sure I was taking my diet seriously too, eating to fuel my body and to keep myself in good shape.

So when the manager, John Yems, asked if I would like to sign for the club, I didn't need to think twice. On 10 January 2021, I walked out onto the pitch and made my professional debut for Crawley Town against Leeds United. I'm very proud to call myself a Crawley player. Life is so short and I urge you to fight for what makes you happy, take chances, change (if change is needed) and don't let anybody tell you you CAN'T, because I'm telling you that with the right mindset and a healthy body and lifestyle, you CAN. My job might tell a different story, but I'm really just a normal guy who balances social life with exercise and good food. I don't just eat salad leaves for lunch or spend three hours a day in the gym. I work out five times a week, I eat healthy home-cooked meals most of the time, but enjoy a Chinese with the missus on a Saturday night, and beers and a burger with my mates when we watch football. My lifestyle isn't abnormal or unachievable and I've loved being able to share that.

I've not chosen to tell you my story for any other reason than to remind you that YOU have a story. You have a journey and you can draw on those experiences, those failures and those successes to remind yourself that you can make positive changes, no matter how hard it seems. Before we go on, I want you to think about those defining moments in your life and use them to give you that push to get fitter, get healthier and get happier, on this new journey.

LIVE
WRIGHT

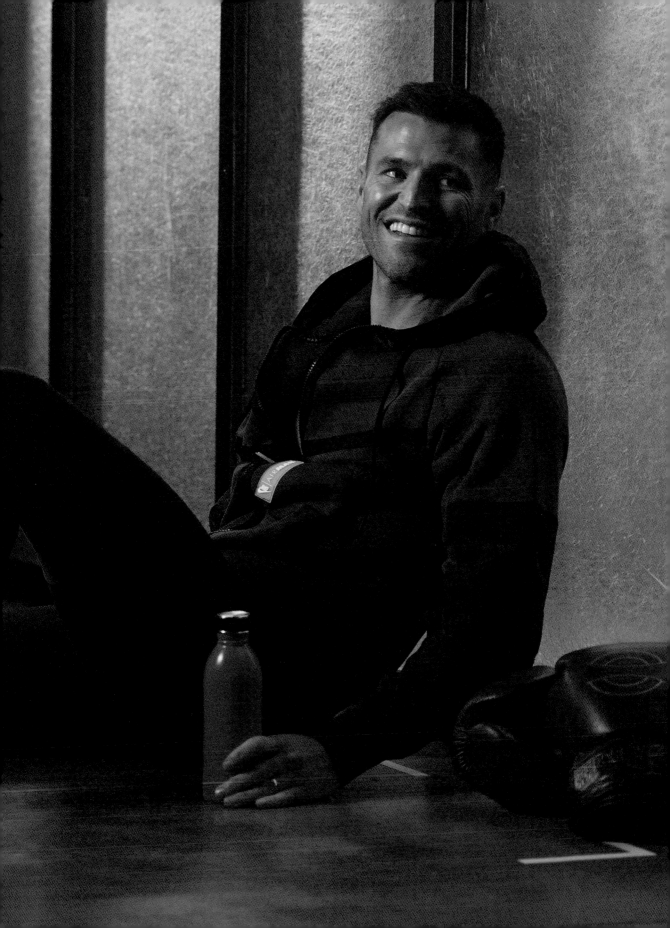

CHAPTER 2 – MY PHILOSOPHY

I'm only in my thirties, but the ups and downs in my life and the crazy road that has led me to this moment have taught me more about the importance of leading a balanced life than I could ever have imagined. At every significant moment, I prioritised what I thought was the most important thing at that particular time and, instead of weighing that up with other things in my life, I just put every single bit of energy into that one thing. I almost binged on it to the point where everything else just got completely neglected. Every time I did this I would achieve what I set out to do, but wonder why I either couldn't sustain it, or wasn't happy once I'd got it.

I've overworked myself – taking on multiple jobs while trying to be a professional football player and not giving my all to any of them – and sacrificed sleep and a good diet, and completely burnt out.

- **I've overindulged, giving myself a whole summer of bingeing on junk food, drinking alcohol and partying, without thinking about the toll that would take on me – both physically and mentally – and, ultimately, how it would ruin my career in professional football.**

- **I've undereaten in many different ways. When I was younger it was by accident while overworking myself and not making time to eat. In the Jungle it was forced upon me. And later in life, for a very short period, I have purposefully undereaten, thinking I was being healthy by watching my calories, but not realising I wasn't eating enough to sustain a healthy body. All three times left me feeling irritable, unproductive, exhausted and not healthy or happy.**

- **I've not prioritised exercise. The first time was during that summer abroad when I let everything go, the second was when I threw all my efforts into work. Every time I've left exercise off my 'to-do list' I have suffered physically and mentally from the lack of movement in my life.**

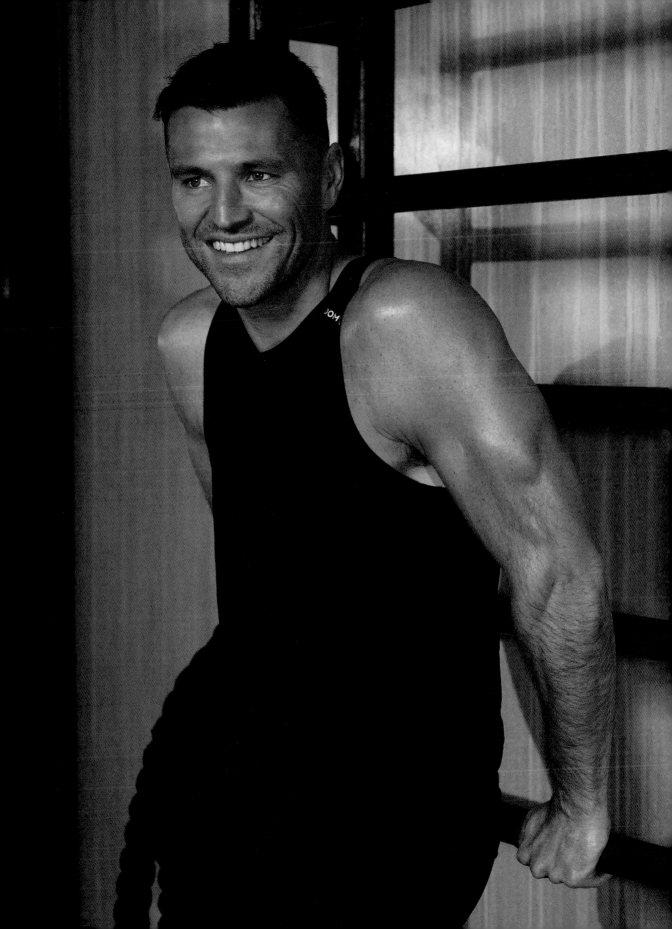

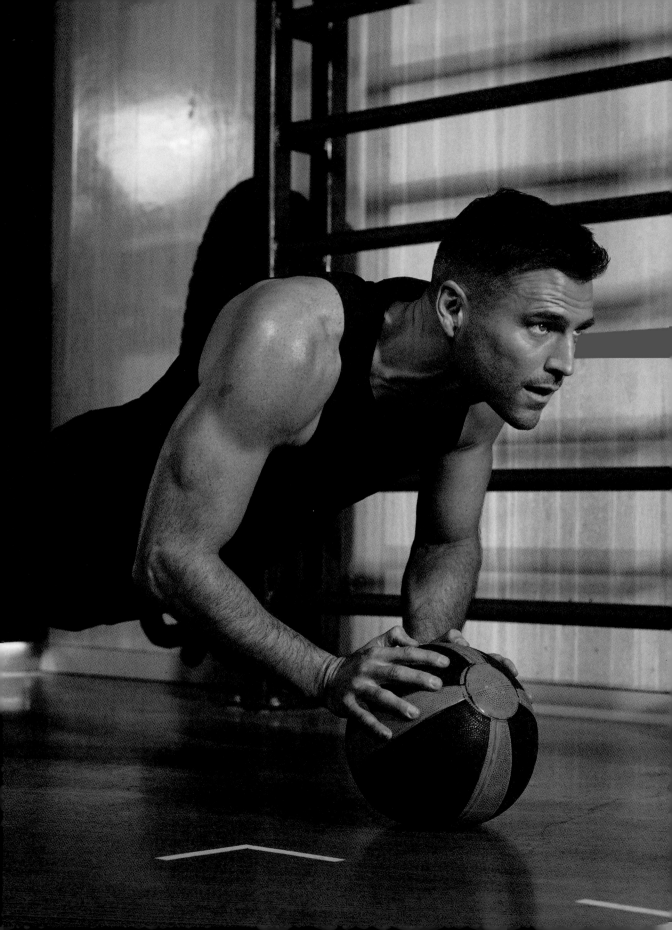

- **I've not prioritised sleep on more occasions than I can bear to mention. For years sleep was something I didn't understand the power of. When I was overworking myself I thought it was an achievement to get by on three hours a night. When I was partying I thought it was cool to stay up all night and even until recently, when I've taken on too much work and wanted to fit in exercise and a social life, I've let sleep be the first thing that is sacrificed. Not only does this impact how I feel, it also negatively impacts how I eat and how I train, all of which I will go into in more detail in this chapter.**

What I'm showing you here is that I wasn't born with motivation to exercise regularly or the ability to understand the importance of a healthy diet and lifestyle. I've learnt it the hard way, by making the mistakes that we all make along the way. I'm sure that, reading this, you are realising you have either done the same, or are doing the same right now. All I have done over the years is reflect. Every time I've failed at something, I've asked myself, 'Why didn't that work out?' And every time it's been because I've let something slip in my lifestyle that has impacted everything else.

It's taken a lot of mistakes to get here, but what I know is that I've learnt from all of them and for the last five years or so, I've been able to bring them all together and to be the fittest, healthiest and, most importantly, the happiest I have ever been. And I can't wait to share how I did this, because once you understand the three pillars of this way of living, it will all fall into place.

I really believe that the most important strength I'm giving you in this book isn't in the workouts, but in the knowledge. You only get one crack at the whip – life is so short – and you don't want to look back and think, 'What if?'

Go for everything, chase your dreams, be who you want to be and don't let anybody tell you any different. But most importantly, do not fear failure. Failure is great. It's the biggest learning curve you could ask for.

Soaking up this chapter and truly understanding what a healthy lifestyle looks like will empower you to want to make the necessary changes to balance out YOUR life.

THE GET FIT, GET HEALTHY, GET HAPPY CYCLE

I'm a visual learner, so I wanted to simplify all these words into a nice, easy, graphic.

Not one of these things is any more important than the other because, as the graphic shows, the minute you let one of these go, the circuit is broken. Of course, no one is perfect and you can't do all of these things in a perfect balance every single day, but over the course of six weeks, you need to make sure you prioritise each of these things and not place all your efforts in just one or two.

To give one example: If I made time for 30 minutes of exercise every day, cooked myself healthy meals and was in bed at the right time to get my eight hours of sleep, that's all great, but what's the point in doing this every day if I'm not making time to see my friends, or family, or spending enough time with my wife?

Some days I'll still do my 30 minutes of exercise, I'll still get my eight hours of sleep, but I'll also go down the pub with my friends, have a few beers and order a burger, because I know how important that is to my mental health.

To give another example: If I get eight hours of sleep every night and hang out with my friends and family but order a takeaway every night, I know that I'm going to feel sluggish, I'm not going to have the right fuel to train, so my exercise is going to suffer – and then my sleep is going to be disrupted too.

It's all about noticing patterns in your lifestyle and recognising when you might be starting to let one, or two, or three healthy habits slip away.

Welcome to your Get Fit, Get Healthy, Get Happy cycle.

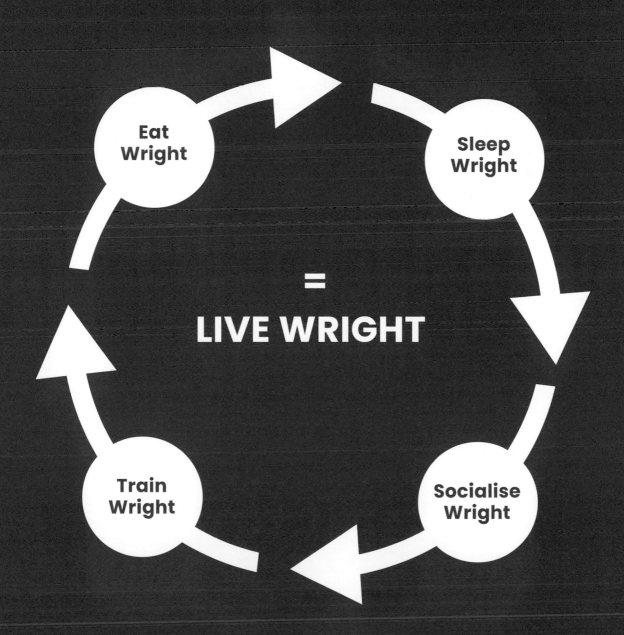

HOW TO GET THE WRIGHT MINDSET

Right guys, here's your first exercise, and it doesn't include a squat or a burpee. I want you to grab a pen and fill in this page. This task only works if you are really honest with yourself. If you struggle to think of what to write down, think back over the last few days or weeks, and see if you can pick things out, or set the book down and spend the next few days noticing your habits, then come back to this page later and fill it in. Remember, this isn't for anyone else but YOU, and getting this bit right before you start could be the difference between making it to the end of the book and giving up halfway through.

Which healthy habits do you prioritise?

(Cooking healthy food, socialising with friends, spending time with the kids, exercising...)

....

Which healthy habits do you let slip?

(Cooking healthy food, socialising with friends, exercising, sleep...)

....

What are your main reasons for letting healthy habits slip?

(Label these barriers from 1–5, 1 being the biggest barrier for you, 5 being the smallest)

Time Energy Motivation Money Responsibilities

Now you've completed this page, take a second to read back over what you've written and really take it in. You should be able to clearly see what aspects of your lifestyle are already healthy, and which could be changed to make for a healthier cycle. Just simply seeing it here, in black and white, will help you understand why you might have struggled in the past, and how to change that for the future.

Here are a few questions to ask yourself for each barrier:

Time
— Could you set your alarm to wake you up 30 minutes earlier a few times a week?
— Could you use half of your lunch break to go for a walk?
— Could you be better at planning ahead?
— Could you move in the advert breaks of your favourite TV show?

Energy
— Are you getting enough sleep?
— Are you eating too much sugar?
— Could you get more variety in your diet?
— Are you drinking enough water?

Motivation
— Have you reminded yourself why you are doing it?
— Are you choosing exercises that you ENJOY?
— Are you rewarding yourself for your efforts?

Money
— Are you overspending on expensive gym memberships you are not using?
— Have you tried bulk cooking and freezing meals to cut costs?
— Are you planning ahead enough?
— Have you used your local outdoor space?

Responsibilities
— Could you walk/cycle to your work or children's school?
— Could you make your social time an active time? E.g. walking coffee meet-up, playing an outdoor game with your kids.
— Have you given yourself a flexible routine?

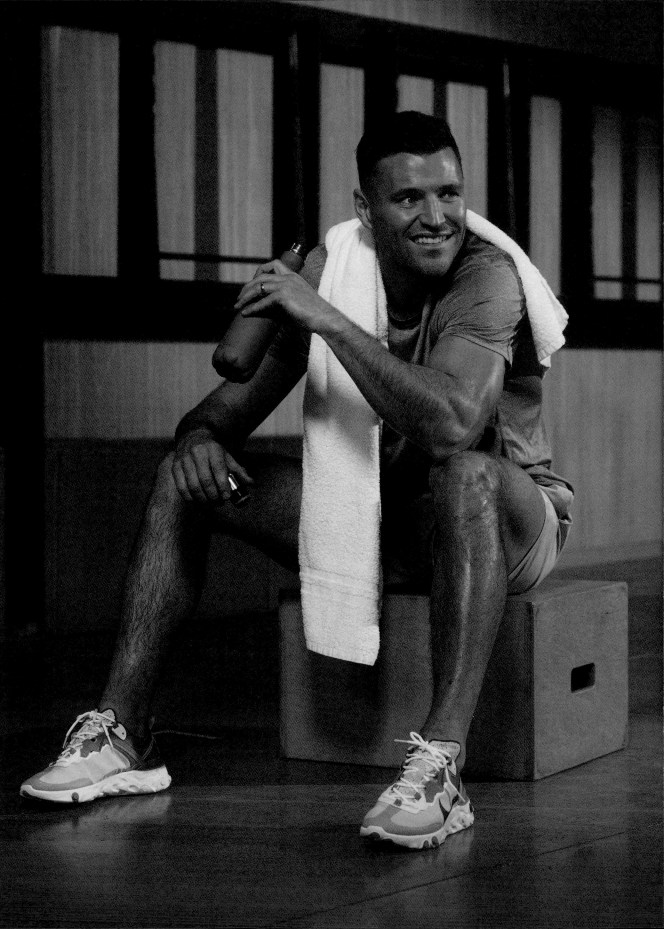

FINDING – AND KEEPING – MOTIVATION

No one is just born with an unlimited amount of motivation, as much as it might seem like it.

Motivation takes work and practice, and everyone who seems to have this magical reserve of it has had to find it in some way or another. It is a bugbear of mine when people say to me, 'It's alright for you, you are naturally fit.' Or, 'I wish I could be as motivated as you, it's just not me.' My answer to this is always that no one is naturally fit, or naturally healthy, and no one has motivation written into their DNA. Everyone has to work at it but once you do, you'll realise it was never as hard as your mind told you it was.

I never wake up thinking, 'I can't wait to work out today', but I do wake up thinking 'I can't wait to reap the benefits of my workout today.' And this is something that I want you all to focus on. Motivation fluctuates. Sometimes you'll have a winning streak of two or three weeks, then one day you'll wake up and find yourself searching for reasons why you should work out, or why you should choose a healthy breakfast over a high-calorie one. And that's when you need to be ready and waiting with those reasons, to give yourself that reminder of why.

Here are the top reminders I keep tucked away in my mind to keep me motivated

Productivity

I know the difference between a day when I haven't exercised and a day that I have. On days I haven't, I'm more sluggish, find it much more difficult to get started and just don't feel as energised as I do if I've completed a workout. This doesn't just relate to work. It could be how much energy I put into cooking a healthy lunch, or how much more effort I put into my relationship or social time with friends. Fitting exercise into my day changes my output on all these things and that's why it's so important to make time to fit it in.

Confidence

Let's be honest – along with how it makes us feel, exercise and eating healthily can also help us to look good too. Whether that's losing weight, toning up or building muscle, when you have completed a workout or exercise, knowing you are contributing to looking a way that makes you feel good is a huge motivating factor. When you feel confident it impacts so many other aspects of your life, whether it's nailing that presentation for work or feeling more confident in the bedroom... feeling good about how you look is something to remember when you are struggling to find motivation.

Health

We all want to take care of our health and, now more than ever, we know that our weight and lifestyle choices directly impact our immunity and lifelong health. We can't 100 per cent prevent every disease and illness that might come our way, but science shows that being fitter and having a healthy weight gives us a much better fighting chance. Remembering that every workout or healthy meal or good night's sleep is contributing to better health is a huge motivator to keep you going.

Happiness

When people see my workout posts or a topless photo of me they can be quick to judge my lifestyle. Even some of my friends say to me, 'Yeah, you look good, but I'm way happier than you because I eat what I want and don't force myself to work out.'

My reply is, 'Bulls***.'

I know that fitting in a 30-minute workout five times a week and eating healthily makes me happier than if I was ordering a takeaway every night and sitting in front of the TV all day.

Of course I still enjoy the odd pizza or curry night every now and then, but I don't do this every day, and I genuinely believe that makes me savour it and enjoy it so much more. Movement and a balanced diet makes me feel good and that directly impacts my happiness.

MY MOTIVATION TIPS

Along with these mental reminders, there are small, day-to-day things I do to give myself that little kick towards making healthier choices. Try giving them a go.

- **Always have healthy snacks on hand**
When a pang of hunger hits us, it is so easy to give in to temptation and reach for an unhealthy option if there isn't an obvious healthy alternative. I always make sure I've got healthy snacks in the house or in my rucksack when I'm out and about. Nuts, fruit, boiled eggs, chopped veg and dips are some of my favourites.

- **'One, two, three, go'**
This is something I do regularly. I know I need to exercise but I'm lying on the sofa and I just can't be bothered to get up. I literally take a deep breath and say to myself, in three seconds I'm going to get up and go work out. I say 'one, two, three' and get my ass up and go and do it.

- **Lay out your kit**
For those who procrastinate in the morning, this one's for you. I always have my gym kit out and ready the night before. It's so easy to get up and just potter around making excuses not to get moving. If you kit is there ready, it's one less excuse. Put your exercise clothes on first thing in the morning, even if you don't plan to work out straight away. This way, if you have a small gap in your day (baby is asleep, a work meeting is cancelled) you are dressed and ready to go.

- **Plan ahead**
My weeks are often very different, so on a Sunday I look at my schedule and plan my exercise and meals so I know when I need to set aside time.

- **Buddy up**
If I'm struggling, I'll draft in help from friends. Whether that's inviting them over to mine for a workout, or even just telling my wife the night before that I'm going to get up and go for a run the next day. Involving other people makes you accountable and drives you to see things through.

- **Line up banging playlists**
Sometimes just knowing I've got a cracking playlist lined up, or a podcast I really want to listen to, will help get me excited about exercise. Spend some time finding yours.

- **Little boosts**
Another simple but effective tool is treating yourself. A new gym tee, a takeaway frothy coffee post workout, or even telling yourself you'll buy that new pair of headphones once you've done 10 workouts. These little rewards can end up being a big boost.

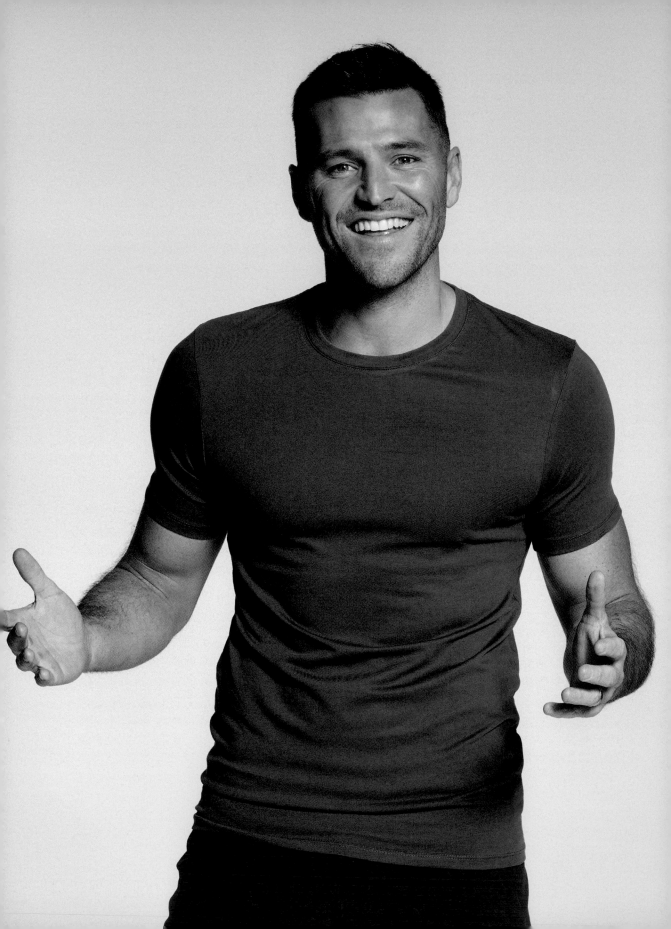

CHAPTER 3 –
HOW TO GET STARTED

BE PREPARED

So much of our success in life comes from being prepared for the unknown. And if 2020 has taught us anything, it's that we can never fully know what's around the corner. What we can do is set ourselves up as best as possible for whatever is coming our way. So let's break it down. To SET ourselves up for a healthy lifestyle, we need to think about those three main pillars:

 Sleep **Eat** **Train**

This book is your guide to living a healthy lifestyle, but to kickstart new exercise and diet habits, I have put together a six-week plan for you to get stuck into. The plan is my way of showing you how to structure exercise plans into your week, how to fit healthier meal choices into a busy lifestyle, and how it will all come together to leave you feeling happier and healthier as a result.

Each week I will take you through four high-intensity workouts, each lasting between 25 and 30 minutes. I also introduce you to LISS (Low Intensity Steady State) training days and two planned rest days. Alongside your new exercise plan, I have put together my favourite recipes so you can learn the beauty of quick, easy, healthy – and delicious – cooking. Choose three meals a day and you'll be eating your way to better sleep, impressive workout energy and positive physical results, in no time.

Every week will throw up different obstacles that could get in the way of achieving the optimum sleep, eating healthy meals or training regularly. This is life. But if we SET ourselves up for success as much as we can, the probability of achieving our goals is so much higher than if we leave it up to chance.

Now you've learnt the route to finding your motivation to get fit, get healthy and get happy, it is important to nail down those goals. You will undoubtedly reach points in the plan where your motivation wavers a little; that's fine, and more than normal, believe me. So if you set out those reasons for why you are going to do it now, they are going to be there when we need them later. Come up with your own, or choose from a list of my favourites:

'I want to feel more confident in all aspects of my life'
'I want to improve my health and live longer'
'I want to be more productive at work/in life'
'I want to lose weight to look and feel better'
**'I want to improve my mood and get out of a
 negative mindset'**
'I want to be a good example for my kids'

PLAN WRIGHT

Now that you have your reasons for committing to a healthy lifestyle locked into your mind, you are well on the way to achieving those goals. The next thing to do is think about how my workouts and meals are going to best fit into your life. I like to train in the morning because I have really busy days and I don't often know when I'll finish or whether I'll have time to fit in exercise once I've left the house. But it's no good me telling you to do the same when we know we are all very different. Take a second now to think about what times of the day work best for you. It might be that it is the same time every day, or it might be that it changes from week to week. Taking time to think about it now can take any stress – or excuses – out of the way later. Opposite is an empty grid to help you pencil in any regular commitments you already have so you can see where you have time to fit in a workout – remember, it's only 30 minutes – or time to cook or prepare a meal.

MONDAY

TUESDAY

WEDNESDAY

THURSDAY

FRIDAY

SATURDAY

SUNDAY

SLEEP WRIGHT

For years I didn't realise how important sleep was. How wrong was I. Over the last few years sleep has finally been given a bit of a platform and the experts have been filling us in on just how crucial it is. Sleep has a direct impact on our physical and mental health. And if you're not convinced sleeping more is going to make you fitter and healthier, here's the lowdown on shut-eye.

Sleep and exercise

When we work out, our body works hard to make physical changes that will improve our muscle strength and our cardiovascular health, but to be able to do this, we have to sleep long enough and well enough so that we can achieve the benefits. Put simply, you could smash out the hardest workout of your life and eat healthy meals, but if you are not getting enough sleep, your body won't be able to deliver results, and you'll end up getting frustrated as to why. If you don't prioritise sleep as much as you prioritise exercise, it's the same as planting thousands of seeds but never watering them. Also, if you aren't getting enough sleep, the chances are you are going to find it a lot harder to find the motivation to work out or put your all into your training, as you'll be constantly battling against tiredness.

Sleep and diet

When we are trying to eat a healthy diet, one thing that can massively impact our success is sleep. If you do not get enough sleep – at least seven hours a night – the hormones that control your hunger levels are impacted. Studies show that people who do not get enough sleep have bigger appetites during the day and find it harder to reach a stage where they feel full, meaning they are much more likely to overeat. Research has also shown that the more sleep-deprived you are, the more likely you are to crave high-sugar, high-calorie foods. I know I find myself wanting chocolate and sweets when I've lost out on sleep. So, the minute you allow your sleep to fall off the priority list, you are setting yourself up to fail when it comes to healthy eating.

To get you started, here are the things I do to improve my sleep:

- **Avoid screens**
  I know it's tempting to get into bed and have a few final scrolls of social media, but switching off from screens at least 30 minutes before going to sleep can really help to turn the mind from 'wide awake' to 'ready for bed'. I have to be strict with myself, but sometimes I'll even leave my phone in another room a few hours before I go to bed to break the habit.

- **Calm breathing**
  I'm not into long meditation sessions or anything too 'zen', but I do know that if I take some good deep breaths when I'm in bed, it helps me take my mind off other things and slows everything down. Try breathing in deeply for four seconds, then out slowly for five seconds and repeat for a minute.

- **Switch off bright lights**
  I try to turn down the lights a good hour or so before going to bed. Switching the main lights off in the living room and putting lamps on instead, or having the bedside light on while I get ready for bed tells my mind that it's wind-down time.

- **Limit food and drink intake**
  If you are struggling to get off to sleep, it might be worth looking at your evening eating habits. Eating too close to bedtime could mean you are too full to feel like drifting off. Also, think about what you are eating. Anything high in sugar or caffeine could be keeping you awake if consumed in the evening.

- **Tidy your room**
  Sometimes it could be as simple as having a tidy bedroom. Getting into bed with a room that is in order can help you feel more calm and ready to switch off. I know that I sleep better if I've put things away and the bedroom isn't a mess.

- **Plan the next day**
  Do this before you get into bed. Something I used to be terrible for was getting into bed and then starting to think about what I was doing the next day. It would set my mind racing and I'd take ages to drift off. If you can, make time after dinner or during a TV advert break to make a list or a plan of what you're doing the next day or annoying chores you've got to do. It will help to stop them keeping you awake at night.

- **Exercise**
  A perfect reason to keep on top of your training. Regular exercise helps us to sleep better. Moving more will help us release hormones, tire out our muscles and get us into a routine. Get up and get moving every day.

Sleep and the mind

Scientific studies have found there is a close relationship between our sleep and our mental health. Poor sleep can have a negative impact on how our mind works. When we are not getting enough shut-eye our chances of feeling anxious, stressed, irritable, lonely, unproductive and low in mood are massively increased.

How to sleep Wright

As I said, I had to completely change my mindset on sleep, from minimal sleeping to 'get by' to maximum sleeping to support a healthy lifestyle. At first I found it difficult to change my routine, but my main advice is to start small and don't put too much pressure on yourself. I aim for between seven and eight hours a night, as this is proven to be the right amount for recovery and rest and I know I feel great on this amount. With only one in three of us (32 per cent) getting seven hours sleep a night, chances are you might be falling below the amount you should be aiming for.

LET'S TALK ABOUT SEX

You love it, I love it, who doesn't love it? Even when you are biting into that incredible chocolate brownie and telling everyone, 'This is better than sex', you know you're lying. Now, you might be thinking, what is a section on sex doing in a health and fitness book, but for me, this is exactly where this chat belongs. Sex is such an important part of life, whether we are in a relationship or not – and having a healthy sex life can massively improve our happiness.

Whether you use this as a motivational tool or something to add into your 'be prepared' mindset, here's my list of reasons why following a healthy lifestyle can lead to better sex – and better sex can lead to a fitter, healthier, happier life.

- Higher sex drive

We know that exercise increases our heart rate and improves blood flow, and that improved blood flow can work wonders for your sex drive. Exercise also releases feel-good endorphins and helps to reduce stress levels. This lovely little concoction massively helps to improve our sex drive.

- Better in bed

This doesn't take too much explaining. The fitter you are, the more stamina you will have both during a workout and in the bedroom. Stronger muscles are also proven to make some people experience more pleasurable sex.

- Confidence boost

Let's face it, no one feels sexy when they are lacking body confidence. Feeling strong, fit and confident in your own skin means you're going to be way more likely to feel good naked. Regular exercise and a nutritious diet can really help boost your mood and how you feel about yourself, and if you feel sexy, chances are your partner is going to notice...

- Less lethargic

No one is in the mood for sex when they feel tired and sluggish. An unhealthy diet of ultra-processed foods and a lack of movement in your day can leave you struggling with this 'fog' of tiredness. A nutritious diet and regular movement will see you snap out of this slump and completely change your mental state in days.

- Closer relationship

If you do have a partner, living a healthier lifestyle can massively benefit your relationship. A nutritious diet and regular exercise is proven to make us less irritable, less stressed and less likely to suffer mood swings and, let's be honest, the first person to benefit from this change is your partner. It's always worth remembering that making a positive change for you is also usually making a positive change for your partner too.

- Better sex = better workouts

Bear with me here, but having a better sex life can actually make us fitter, healthier and happier.

- Having sex boosts serotonin, our happy hormone

This improves our mood and can even help fight off depression and anxiety.

- Improved sleep

Regular sex also helps us sleep better.

EAT WRIG

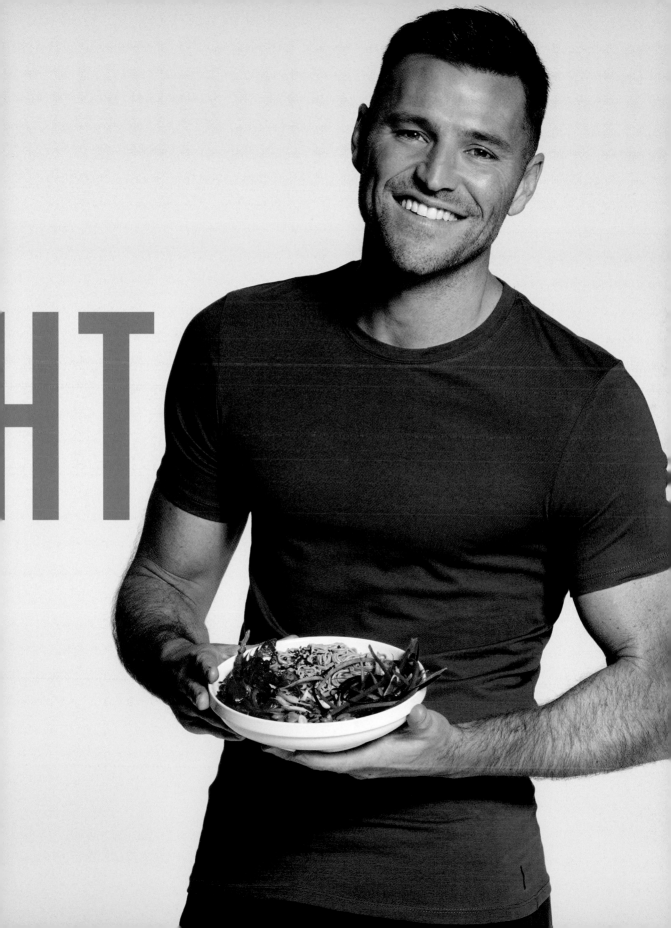

HT

CHAPTER 4 – GET COOKING

I have always had a big appetite. To me, food is just pure enjoyment, which is why my friends say I'm a 'fat boy waiting to break out.' The reason I tell you this is because I want to make something clear really early on: NEVER GO HUNGRY. 'Diet plan' doesn't mean starving yourself or missing out on the food you love. I want you to see your diet as an exciting part of this journey in which you will reap the benefits of balancing the healthy with the less-healthy.

My wife Michelle introduced me to so many different ways to eat healthily – swapping regular pasta for gluten-free and incorporating more fish into my diet. She's an amazing cook and it opened my eyes to the ways you can bring more flavour and texture into food. I've blended her cooking skills with my favourite cuisines, to bring you recipes that are dinner-party worthy, without hours of effort.

What I've learnt about food
- **Healthy eating doesn't mean going hungry**
- **Healthy eating doesn't mean boring food**
- **Healthy eating doesn't mean expensive ingredients**
- **Healthy eating doesn't mean spending hours in the kitchen**

THE RECIPE PLAN

All of the recipes here are nutritionally varied and quick and easy to cook, each providing a daily average calorie intake of around 1,800 kcals, helping you to fuel your body but also achieve steady weight loss. All the meals have hearty portion sizes, to help you get great results without battling hunger or suffering a lack of energy. If you follow the plan, you should eat three meals, choosing one from Breakfasts, one from Lunch and one from Dinner, along with one from Snacks. You can consume black coffee, herbal tea and water alongside these meals.

Variation
Some recipes have variations, but be aware that changing ingredients alters the calorie count. 'Optional' ingredients are not in the calorie count.

MY FOOD TIPS

Don't overcook your veg
Burning your veg, or even just overcooking it, is bad news from a nutritional perspective. Cook them too much and all those minerals that are going to nourish your mind and body are destroyed, leaving you with less of the good stuff.

Use smaller plates
Lots of us have been taught that we should always finish everything on our plates, but portion control is key to building healthier habits with food. Try not to use huge plates when serving up your meals, as the temptation to overfill them will see you dishing up more calories than you need. Using smaller plates will help you manage your portions.

Always have healthy snacks in the house/with you
Snacking is normal, and if you are to stick to my 'never go hungry' mantra then there will be times that you just need to eat something in between meals. The problem arises when you have nothing healthy to reach for at these times. Make sure you have veg, nuts, berries, olives – anything high in protein and low in sugar and carbs – to keep you going and prevent you reaching for crisps and biscuits.

Take your time
If you are anything like me, you are used to doing things at a million an hour. But one thing I take my time over is eating. Sit down and enjoy your food at a slow pace. Not only will you give your body time to properly digest what you are eating, you will also really appreciate the food and be much more likely to pay attention to when you are full than if you rush it.

Hydrate
The importance of staying hydrated throughout the day is huge, not only to keep the systems in your body working properly, but also to prevent yourself from confusing hunger with thirst. Before reaching for a snack, try drinking water first to see if you need to quench your thirst. I also advise drinking water with your meal rather than flavoured drinks.

Prep
We don't always have time to cook, but prepping food ahead of time can be a game changer when trying to eat well. On days when you have more time, cook up double quantities of a recipe then freeze half ready for that day when you just don't have time to pull a healthy meal together. You could also pre-chop veg and freeze it, to cut down preparation time for future meals.

BREAKFAS

ON-THE-GO OAT AND CRANBERRY BREAKFAST BARS

Makes: 12 bars
Prep: 15 minutes
Cook: 15–20 minutes

250g (9oz/2½ cups) rolled oats
75g (3oz/½ cup) chopped
    hazelnuts
150g (5oz/generous 1 cup) dried
    cranberries
2 tsp ground cinnamon
grated zest of 1 orange, plus
    2 tbsp juice
120ml (4fl oz/½ cup) sunflower
    oil, plus extra for brushing
6 tbsp clear honey
2 tbsp soft brown sugar

PER BAR:

330 KCALS

3.4g PROTEIN

17g FAT

22g CARBS

Make these quick and easy bars at the weekend and you're well supplied for the week ahead. The oats supply protein and fibre as well as slow-release energy to prevent spikes in your blood sugar levels. What's more, they're heart-healthy and help lower cholesterol. And because these bars are made with vegetable oil, not butter, they don't contain saturated fat.

1. Preheat the oven to 180°C (160°C fan/350°F/gas 4). Lightly brush a 20 x 20cm (8 x 8in) baking tin with oil and line with baking parchment.
2. Put the oats, hazelnuts, cranberries, cinnamon and orange zest in a bowl.
3. Heat the oil, honey and sugar in a small saucepan over a low heat, stirring until the sugar dissolves. Mix into the oat mixture with the orange juice. If the mixture is too dry, add a little water; if it's not firm enough and is too sticky, add more oats.
4. Spoon into the prepared tin and smooth the top, pressing down with the back of a metal spoon to level it out. Bake in the preheated oven for 15–20 minutes, or until firm and golden brown.
5. Cool slightly before cutting into 12 bars. Leave in the tin until completely cold, then remove and store in an airtight container.

Or try this...
• Add some dark chocolate chips or mixed seeds.
• Instead of hazelnuts use walnuts or flaked almonds.
• Use maple syrup or agave syrup instead of honey.

SPEEDY HOMEMADE BIRCHER MUESLI

Serves 2
Prep: 15 minutes
Soak: at least 1 hour, or overnight

4 tbsp unsweetened apple juice
250g (9oz/generous 1 cup)
   natural or vanilla low-fat
   yoghurt, plus 2 tbsp for topping
100g (3½oz/1 cup) jumbo
   porridge oats
2 red apples, cored and chopped
   or thinly sliced
2 tbsp chopped almonds or
   hazelnuts
1 tbsp dried cranberries

PER SERVING:
410 KCALS
14.5g PROTEIN
11.2g FAT
61g CARBS

You can make your own muesli in a few minutes, and it's cheaper and healthier than buying it. Porridge oats are the perfect breakfast because they're low-GI (glycaemic index) carbs. Your body breaks them down slowly, so your blood sugar levels rise gradually, helping you to feel full for longer.

1. Beat the apple juice and yoghurt together in a bowl, and stir in the oats. Set aside in a cool place for at least 1 hour, or even overnight in the fridge, until the oats absorb the yoghurt and soften.
2. Divide between 2 shallow serving bowls and top with the rest of the yoghurt. Put the apples on top and sprinkle with the nuts and cranberries. Serve immediately.

Tip: You can soak the oats in a screw-top jar in the fridge overnight and then add the toppings the following day and take your breakfast to work with you.

Or try this...
• Top with chopped pears, peaches, strawberries, blueberries, raspberries or whatever fruit is in season.
• Sprinkle with coconut flakes or chia seeds.
• Add a spoonful of crunchy peanut butter.

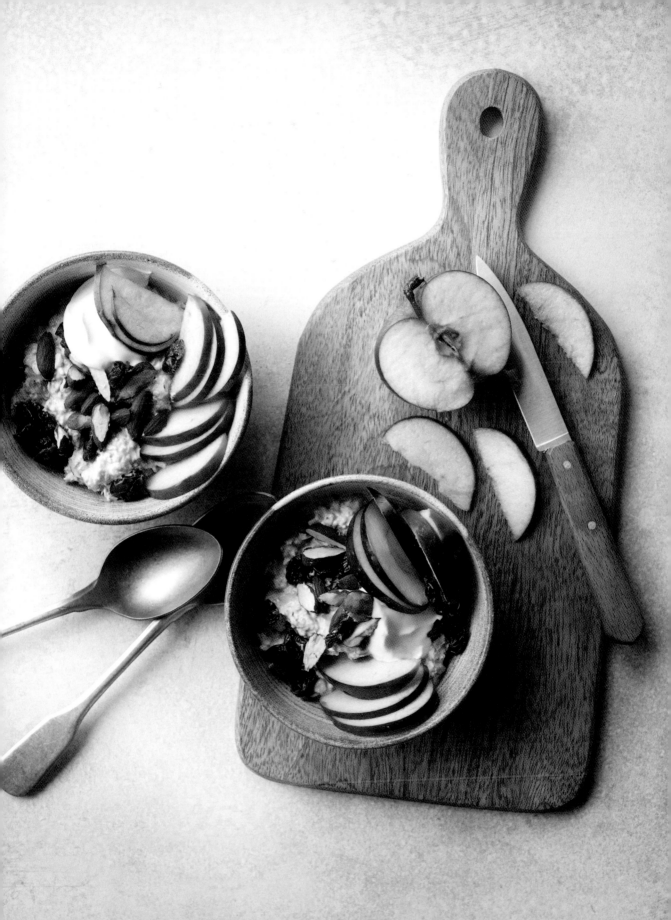

FRUITY CHIA SEED PORRIDGE

Serves 2
Prep: 10 minutes
Chill: overnight

2 ripe medium bananas, mashed
4 tbsp chia seeds
300ml (½ pint/1¼ cups)
    unsweetened coconut
    milk drink
2 drops of vanilla extract
grated zest of 1 orange
4 tbsp coconut yoghurt
100g (3½oz/1 cup) fresh
    blueberries
seeds of ½ pomegranate
    (optional)

Seedy nut sprinkle:
2 tbsp chopped pistachios
1 tbsp sunflower or pumpkin
    seeds
1 tbsp toasted pine nuts

PER SERVING:
390 KCALS
13.6g PROTEIN
18g FAT
49g CARBS

This is such a healthy, nutritious breakfast. Chia seeds are very high in protein, vitamins, minerals, fibre and omega-3 fats, and swell in the coconut milk to make a delicious creamy 'porridge'. Don't use canned coconut milk, which is very high in fat; you want to buy a carton of fresh or long-life unsweetened coconut milk 'drink', which has approximately 20 kcals per 100ml.

1. Put the bananas, chia seeds and coconut milk in a large bowl and whisk until smooth and lump free. Leave to stand for 3 minutes then whisk in the vanilla extract and orange zest. Divide between 2 shallow serving bowls and chill overnight in the fridge.
2. Mix together the ingredients for the seedy nut sprinkle and store in a sealed container.
3. By the following morning the chia mixture should have thickened to a tapioca-like consistency. Top with the yoghurt, blueberries and pomegranate seeds (if using), and scatter the seedy nut sprinkle over the top.

Or try this...
• Use unsweetened almond milk instead of coconut.
• Sprinkle with toasted coconut flakes or some muesli or granola.
• Use different nuts in the sprinkle, such as almonds, walnuts or hazelnuts.
• Add some dried fruit, e.g. cranberries, raisins or goji berries.

SCRAMBLED EGG AND SMASHED AVOCADO TOASTIES

Serves 2
Prep: 5 minutes
Cook: 4–5 minutes

4 medium free-range eggs
1 tbsp skimmed milk
1 ripe avocado, halved, stoned
   and peeled
juice of ½ lime
a few sprigs of parsley or
   coriander, chopped
75g (3oz/⅓ cup) extra light soft
   cheese
2 thick slices wholegrain or
   wholemeal bread
spray olive oil
salt and freshly ground black
   pepper
dried red chilli flakes, for
   sprinkling

PER SERVING:
385 KCALS
24g PROTEIN
23g FAT
17g CARBS

This takes avocado toast into another dimension. Serving it topped with creamy scrambled eggs will boost your protein intake and give you a jackpot of vitamins and minerals to start the day.

1. Beat the eggs and milk in a bowl with some salt and pepper.
2. Coarsely mash the avocado flesh with the lime juice in a bowl and stir in the herbs and soft cheese. Season to taste.
3. Toast the bread and spread the avocado mixture on top.
4. Lightly spray a small non-stick saucepan with oil and place over a low to medium heat. Add the beaten eggs and stir with a wooden spoon until they scramble and start to set. Remove from the heat Immediately.
5. Spoon the scrambled egg over the avocado and sprinkle with the chilli flakes.

Or try this...
• Add some diced tomato to the smashed avocado.
• Use lemon juice instead of lime.
• Serve the scrambled eggs and avocado on grilled giant field or portobello mushrooms instead of toast.
• Use as a filling for warmed wraps or tortillas.

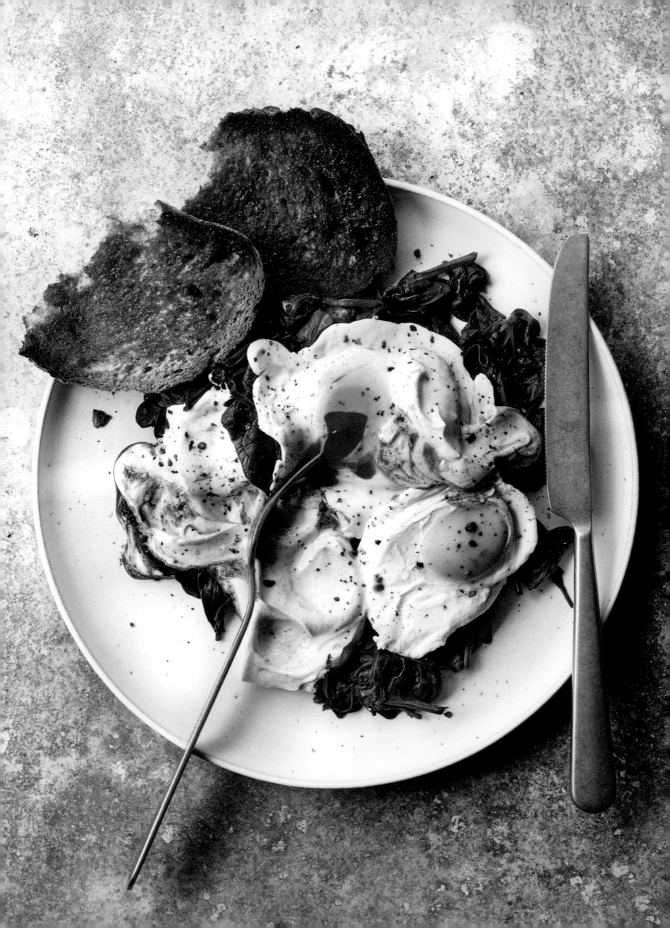

SPICY TURKISH POACHED EGGS

Serves 2
Prep: 10 minutes
Cook: 3–4 minutes

300g (10oz) spinach, trimmed
1 tbsp white wine vinegar
4 medium free-range eggs
250g (9oz/generous 1 cup) 0% fat
 Greek yoghurt
2 garlic cloves, crushed
½–1 tsp harissa paste
2 thick slices wholegrain or
 wholemeal bread or toast
salt and freshly ground black
 pepper

PER SERVING:
345 KCALS
28g PROTEIN
13.5g FAT
26g CARBS

If you feel like a healthy cooked breakfast, you can make this in 15 minutes flat. Basically, it's a simpler and lighter version of eggs Florentine. The spinach really does you good, too – it's jam-packed with vitamins A, C and E as well as iron. Wash it all down with a glass of orange juice to help you absorb the iron and boost your intake.

1. Put the spinach in a large colander. Bring a kettle of water to the boil and pour it over the spinach. When it wilts, press down with a saucer to squeeze out all the excess juice. Season with salt and pepper and keep warm.
2. Bring a pan of water to the boil. Add the vinegar and reduce the heat to a simmer. Carefully crack the eggs one at a time into a bowl, then slide them gently into the simmering water. Poach for 3–4 minutes, or until the whites are set and the yolks are still runny. Remove with a slotted spoon and drain on kitchen paper.
3. Meanwhile, in another pan, heat the yoghurt and garlic over the lowest possible heat to prevent the yoghurt separating. Swirl in the harissa paste.
4. Divide the spinach between 2 bowls and spoon over most of the yoghurt. Add the poached eggs and top with the remaining yoghurt. Serve immediately with the bread or toast. Alternatively, pile everything on top of the toast.

Tip: Harissa is very fiery, so add it a little at a time, tasting as you go.

Or try this...
• If you don't have harissa paste, drizzle the eggs with hot sauce or sprinkle with dried crushed chilli flakes. Or, for a milder flavour, sprinkle with mild Aleppo red pepper flakes or some paprika.
• Instead of toast, serve with wholemeal pitta breads or some English muffins.

ON-THE-GO CHEESY BREAKFAST MUFFINS

Makes 12 muffins
Prep: 15 minutes
Cook: 30–35 minutes

1 tbsp olive oil
1 onion, finely chopped
¼ tsp ground nutmeg
100g (3½oz) baby spinach
   leaves, roughly torn
2 tbsp chopped parsley, chives
   or dill
250g (9oz/2½ cups) self-raising
   flour
1 tsp bicarbonate of soda
a good pinch of salt
2 medium free-range eggs,
   beaten
225g (8oz/1 cup) full-fat Greek
   yoghurt
100g (3½oz/1 cup) grated
   Cheddar cheese, plus extra for
   sprinkling
2 large carrots, grated
3 tbsp seeds, e.g. chia or
   pumpkin

PER MUFFIN:
166 KCALS
7g PROTEIN
6.7g FAT
19g CARBS

Make these muffins in advance and eat a couple on the go when you're in a hurry and don't have time to sit down for breakfast. They freeze well so you could make double the quantity and freeze one batch – just leave them to cool, then seal in freezer bags. A single muffin also makes a tasty snack.

1. Preheat the oven to 200°C (180°C fan/400°F/gas 6) and line a 12-hole muffin tin with paper cases.
2. Heat the oil in a frying pan over a medium heat, cook the onion, stirring occasionally, for 6–8 minutes, or until softened. Stir in the nutmeg and spinach and cook for 1 minute until the leaves turn bright green and wilt. Add the herbs and cool.
3. Sift the flour, bicarbonate of soda and salt into a large mixing bowl.
4. Beat the eggs and yoghurt in a separate bowl then gently fold into the flour with the cooled onion and spinach mixture, grated cheese, carrots and seeds.
5. Divide the mixture evenly among the paper cases and sprinkle lightly with extra grated cheese. Bake in the preheated oven for 20–25 minutes, or until cooked, risen and golden brown.
6. Leave to cool in the tin for a few minutes before transferring the muffins to a wire rack. Eat warm or store in an airtight container for up to 2 days.

Tip: To test whether the muffins are cooked, insert a thin skewer into the centre – it should come out clean.

Or try this...
• Instead of Cheddar, add some diced feta.
• Add some pine nuts or chopped walnuts.
• Add some diced crispy bacon.

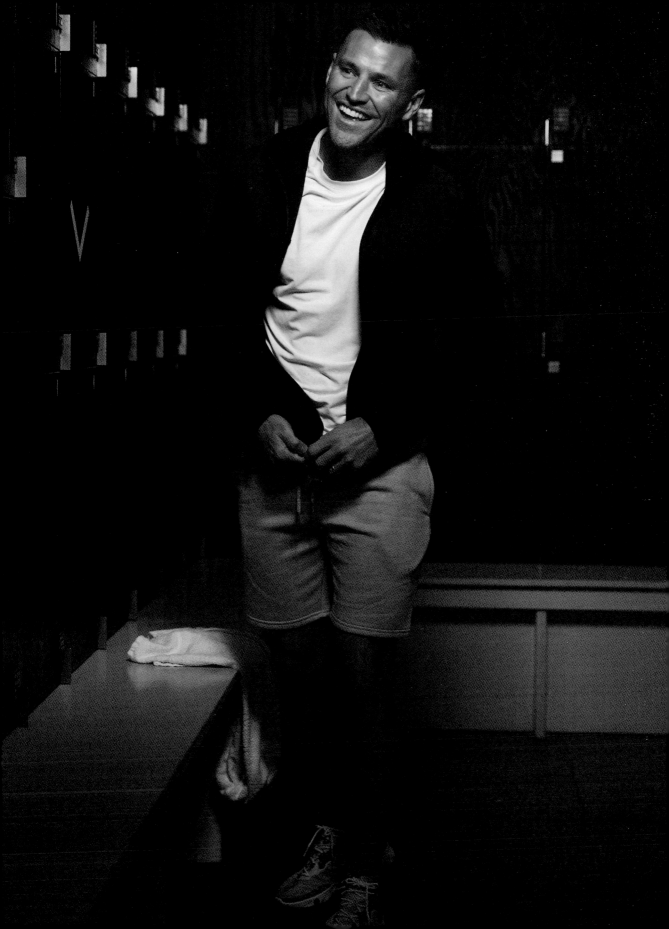

VEGGIE ENGLISH TRAYBAKE BREAKFAST

Serves 2
Prep: 10 minutes
Cook: 15–20 minutes

spray olive oil
4 vegetarian meat-free
   sausages, e.g. Quorn
200g (7oz) open field or chestnut
   mushrooms
200g (7oz) cherry or baby plum
   tomatoes, halved
100g (3½oz) baby spinach leaves
4 medium free-range eggs
50g (2oz/½ cup) grated Cheddar
   cheese
salt and freshly ground black
   pepper

PER SERVING:
360 KCALS
7g PROTEIN
6.7g FAT
19g CARBS

The amazing thing about this veggie breakfast is that everything is cooked in the same tin, so there's practically no washing up afterwards. It fills you up, keeps you going through the morning until lunchtime, and it's really healthy and nutritious. What's not to like?

1. Preheat the oven to 200ºC (180ºC fan/400ºF/gas 6).
2. Lightly spray a large non-stick roasting tin with oil. Add the sausages, mushrooms (open-side down) and tomatoes, and cook for 10–15 minutes in the preheated oven.
3. Meanwhile, put the spinach leaves in a colander and pour some boiling water over them so they wilt and turn bright green. Press down with a saucer and pat dry with kitchen paper to remove any excess moisture.
4. Turn the sausages and mushrooms over and place little heaps of spinach around them in the tin. Make 4 indentations and crack an egg into each one. Season with salt and pepper and sprinkle the cheese over the vegetables.
5. Bake in the oven for about 5 minutes, or until the sausages are cooked, the cheese has melted, and the egg whites are set but the yolks are still runny. Transfer to 2 plates and serve immediately.

Or try this...
• Serve with 4 rashers grilled back bacon.
• Substitute pork sausages for the veggie ones.
• Add some drained canned chickpea or beans with the eggs and cheese.

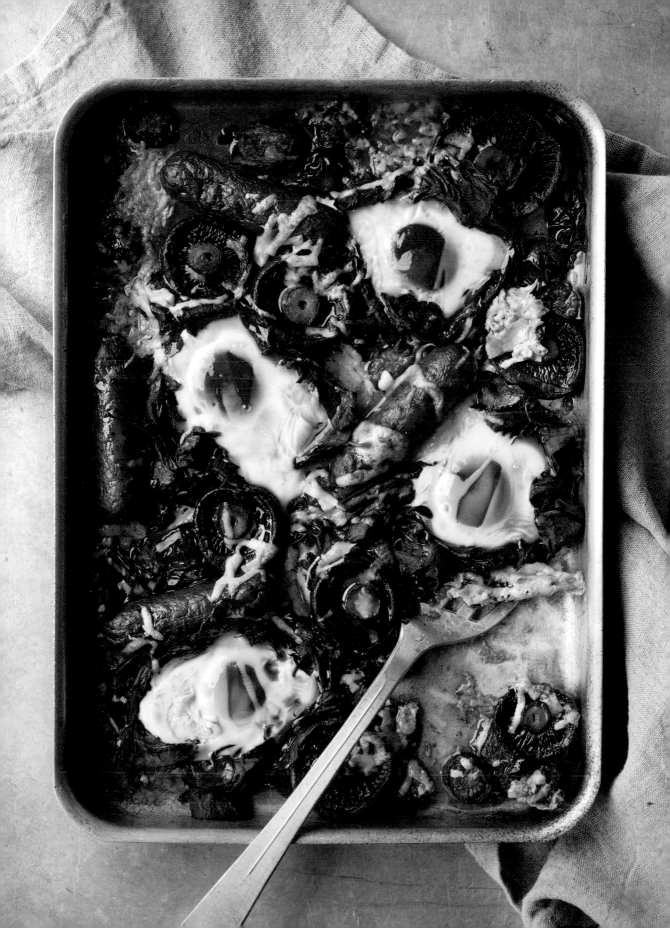

LUNCHES

EASY PEASY CHICKEN MISO SOUP

Serves 4
Prep: 15 minutes
Cook: 25 minutes

2 tbsp olive oil
8 spring onions, sliced
3 garlic cloves, crushed
2.5cm (1in) piece fresh root
  ginger, peeled and diced
2 celery sticks, chopped
400g (14oz) skinned chicken
  breast fillets, thinly sliced
1 red chilli, deseeded and
  shredded
300g (10oz/4 cups) sliced
  shiitake mushrooms
1 litre (33fl oz/generous 4 cups)
  hot chicken stock
4 tbsp white miso paste
250g (9oz) kale or spinach,
  trimmed and shredded
400g (14oz) pre-cooked rice
  noodles
a dash of lime juice
2 tbsp light soy sauce or nam pla
  (Thai fish sauce)
a handful of coriander, chopped,
  to serve

This umami-tasting soup is healthy, cleansing and full of nutritional goodness – it has a whopping 34g protein per serving! And it keeps well in a sealed container in the fridge for a couple of days. If you don't have fresh chicken breasts, it's a great way to use up leftover cooked chicken from the Sunday roast.

1. Heat the oil in a large saucepan over a medium heat. Add the spring onions, garlic, ginger, celery and chicken and cook, stirring occasionally, for 6–8 minutes, or until the vegetables soften and the chicken is golden brown. Add the chilli and mushrooms and cook for 3–4 minutes.
2. Pour in the hot stock and bring to the boil. Reduce the heat to a simmer and add the miso paste, stirring until it dissolves. Cook gently for 10 minutes.
3. Add the kale or spinach and the rice noodles. Simmer for 4–5 minutes then stir in the lime juice and soy sauce or nam pla.
4. Divide the soup among 4 shallow bowls, sprinkle with coriander and serve immediately.

Tip: For the best flavour, make your own stock. Otherwise, use the best-quality stock you can buy.

Or try this...
• For a 'hot and sour' flavour add 1 teaspoon rice vinegar at the end.
• Add some canned sweetcorn, bean sprouts or sugar snap peas.
• Use dark green cabbage, spring greens or Brussels sprout tops.

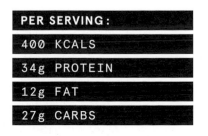

PER SERVING:

400 KCALS

34g PROTEIN

12g FAT

27g CARBS

FRUITY TURKEY MAYO WRAPS

Serves 2
Prep: 15 minutes

2 tbsp light mayonnaise
3 tbsp 0% fat Greek yoghurt
1 tbsp mango chutney
1 small red bird's eye chilli,
   deseeded and diced
a few sprigs coriander or parsley,
   finely chopped
150g (5oz/1½ cups) diced or
   shredded cooked turkey breast
1 small ripe mango, peeled,
   stoned and diced
crisp lettuce leaves, e.g. Cos or
   Little Gem, shredded
2 large wholemeal or wholegrain
   wraps
1 small ripe avocado, peeled,
   stoned and sliced
salt and freshly ground black
   pepper

PER SERVING:
460 KCALS
27g PROTEIN
18.5g FAT
64g CARBS

These yummy wraps are full of goodness and make a delicious packed lunch. You can prepare the turkey mayo the night before and leave it to chill in the fridge. The following morning, before you leave home, assemble the wraps, adding the lettuce and avocado. They're also a great way of using up the Christmas turkey. You can add some cold stuffing, bread sauce or cranberry sauce.

1. Mix together the mayonnaise, yoghurt and chutney in a bowl. Stir in the chilli, chopped herbs, turkey and mango. Season to taste with salt and pepper.
2. Place some lettuce on the wraps, not right up to the edge. Top with the sliced avocado and turkey mayo mixture. Fold or roll the wraps around the filling, and enjoy!

Tip: If you're making the wraps in advance to take to work, lightly brush the avocado with lime or lemon juice to prevent it discolouring.

Or try this...
• Use diced chicken or cooked prawns instead of turkey.
• Use papaya or peaches instead of mango.
• Add some raisins or toasted pine nuts to the turkey mayo mixture.
• Add some sliced tomatoes or bottled roasted red peppers.

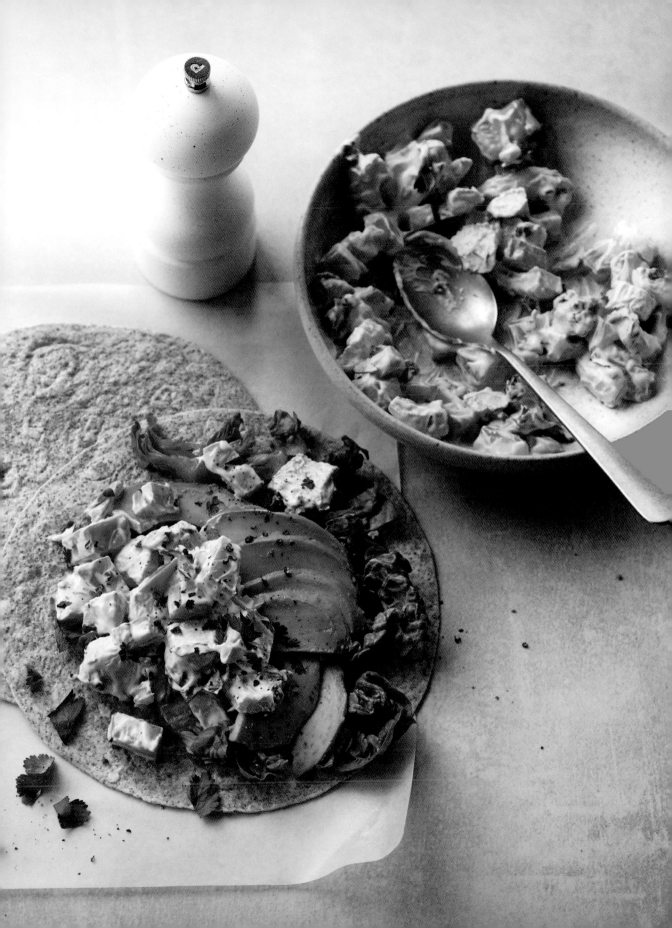

SMOKED SALMON TORTILLA WEDGES

Serves 2
Prep: 10 minutes
Cook: 20 minutes

2 tbsp olive oil
200g (7oz) diced cooked
  potatoes
1 bunch of spring onions, diced
1 garlic clove, crushed
4 medium free-range eggs
a handful of dill, finely chopped
125g (4½oz) smoked salmon,
  diced or cut into strips
45g (1½oz/generous ¼ cup)
  frozen peas
salt and freshly ground black
  pepper

PER SERVING:

480 KCALS
30g PROTEIN
31g FAT
19.6g CARBS

This smoked salmon tortilla is a variation on a traditional Spanish omelette. It's really versatile and you can eat the wedges warm or cold for breakfast, lunch or supper. They are perfect for packed lunches and picnics. And another bonus: you can enjoy a wedge (160 kcals each) as one of your daily snacks.

1. Heat the oil in a large non-stick frying pan over a low to medium heat. Add the potatoes, spring onions and garlic and cook, stirring occasionally, for 5 minutes, or until the potatoes are golden brown and the onions are tender.

2. Meanwhile, beat the eggs in a bowl until foamy then stir in the dill, smoked salmon and peas. Season lightly with salt and pepper.

3. Pour the egg mixture into the hot pan and turn down the heat as low as it can go. Cook very gently for about 10 minutes, or until the tortilla is set and golden brown underneath and the top is starting to set, too.

4. Meanwhile, preheat an overhead grill until it's really hot. Pop the pan underneath the grill for a few minutes, watching it carefully, until the top of the tortilla is set and golden brown.

5. Slide the tortilla out of the pan onto a plate or board and set aside for 5 minutes or so, until it's lukewarm or completely cold, depending on when you want to eat it. Cut into 6 wedges. If you're not eating them immediately, store in a sealed container in the fridge for up to 2 days.

Or try this...
• Use cold poached salmon or flaked hot smoked salmon.
• If you don't have dill, try parsley, chives or even coriander.
• Cook some diced carrot and celery with the potatoes, or add some frozen peas.

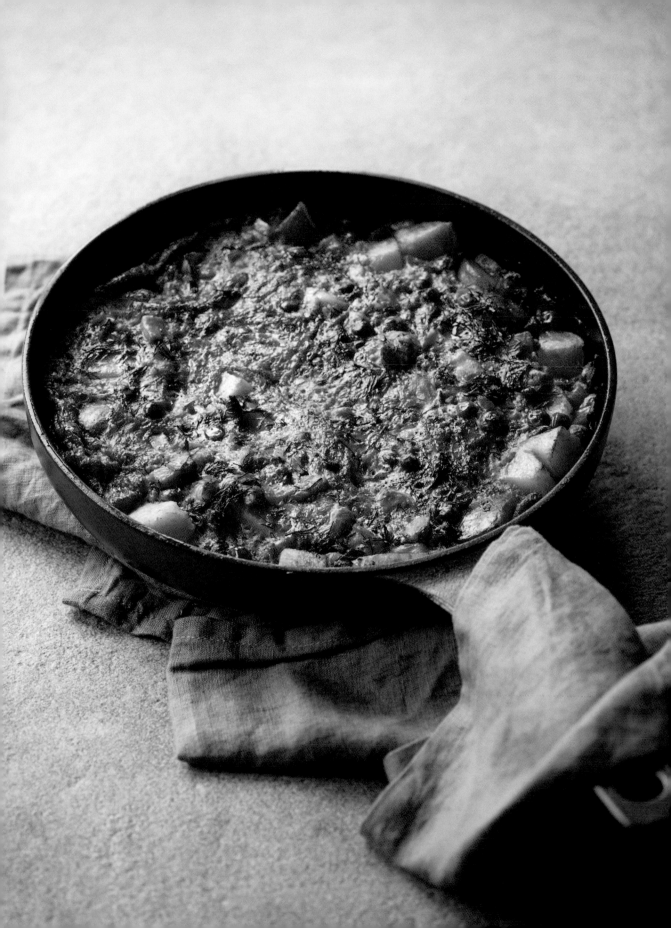

SMOKEY BEANS ON TOAST

Serves 2
Prep: 5 minutes
Cook: 15 minutes

spray olive oil
1 small red onion, finely chopped
1 tsp smoked paprika
1 x 400g (14oz) can chopped
    tomatoes
1 tbsp tomato paste
a pinch of sugar
1 x 400g (14oz) can cannellini
    beans, rinsed and drained
a few drops of balsamic vinegar
4 slices wholemeal or wholegrain
    bread
2 garlic cloves, halved
salt and freshly ground black
    pepper
chopped parsley, to serve

PER SERVING:
390 KCALS
21g PROTEIN
4g FAT
56g CARBS

Homemade beans on toast taste so much better than the readymade canned variety in tomato sauce, and they're full of protein, dietary fibre and vitamins. Plus, you can rustle them up in 20 minutes flat for an easy cooked lunch. Alternatively, make them for breakfast or brunch.

1. Lightly spray a saucepan with oil and set over a low to medium heat. Add the red onion and cook for 5 minutes, stirring occasionally, until softened.
2. Stir in the smoked paprika and cook for 1 minute. Add the tomatoes, tomato paste and sugar, and cook for 5 minutes. Stir in the beans and simmer gently for 5 minutes, or until the sauce has reduced and thickened. Add some balsamic vinegar and salt and pepper to taste.
3. Lightly toast the bread and rub one side of each slice with the cut garlic. Top with the beans, then sprinkle with parsley and serve.

Or try this...
- Add some diced chilli or a dash of Tabasco to the beans.
- Cook 2 crushed garlic cloves with the onion.
- Use canned kidney beans, butter beans or mixed beans instead of cannellini.
- Sprinkle with grated cheese.

TUNA MELT TOASTIES

Serves 2
Prep: 10 minutes
Cook: 4–6 minutes

1 x 160g can tuna in spring water,
   drained
1 small bunch of spring onions,
   finely chopped
a few sprigs of flat-leaf parsley,
   finely chopped
3 tbsp light mayonnaise
50g (2oz/½ cup) grated Cheddar
   cheese
a squeeze of lemon juice
spray olive oil
4 medium slices wholemeal or
   wholegrain bread
salt and freshly ground black
   pepper

PER SERVING:
420 KCALS
33g PROTEIN
17g FAT
27g CARBS

These melt-in-the mouth toasted sandwiches, oozing with cheese, are surprisingly filling. Enjoy them on their own or with a crunchy salad for an easy, nutritious lunch.

1. Put the tuna in a bowl and flake with a fork. Add the spring onions, parsley, mayonnaise, Cheddar and lemon juice and mix until you have a fairly stiff mixture. Season with salt and pepper.
2. Lightly spray one side of each slice of bread with oil. Place 2 slices of bread, oiled side down, on a work surface and divide the tuna mayo mixture between them. Top with the remaining bread, oiled side up and facing outwards.
3. Turn on your sandwich toaster/press and lightly spray the plates with oil. When it's hot, add a sandwich and toast for 4–6 minutes, or until the bread is golden brown and the cheese has melted.
4. Serve the toasties, cut into halves or quarters, and eat them immediately.

Tip: If you don't have a sandwich toaster, cook the toasties in a lightly oiled frying pan for 3–4 minutes each side, or until crisp and golden brown and the cheese melts.

Or try this...
• Use some diced red onion instead of spring onions.
• Add some diced celery or grated carrot to the tuna mayo.
• Add a couple of drops of balsamic vinegar instead of lemon juice.

EASY BEAN MINESTRONE

Serves 4
Prep: 20 minutes
Cook: 35 minutes

2 tbsp olive oil
1 large onion, finely chopped
2 carrots, diced
2 celery sticks, diced
2 garlic cloves, crushed
2 large potatoes, peeled and
   diced
2 courgettes, diced
2 tomatoes, skinned and
   chopped
1.2 litres (2 pints/5 cups) hot
   vegetable stock
a pinch of dried oregano
2 x 400g (14oz) cans butterbeans,
   rinsed and drained
200g (7oz) baby spinach leaves
a handful of flat-leaf parsley,
   chopped
4 tbsp grated Parmesan cheese
salt and freshly ground black
   pepper

Chilli oil:
4 tsp fruity green olive oil
1 tsp dried crushed red chilli
   flakes

I like to make a big pan of soup at the weekend, so I have lots on hand to reheat for lunch or a light supper on busy weekdays when there's no time to cook. It's packed with vegetables and a great way to get your five-a-day, too.

1. Make the chilli oil: mix the oil and chilli flakes together and set aside while you make the soup.
2. Heat the oil in a large saucepan over a medium heat. Add the onion, carrots, celery and garlic and cook, stirring occasionally, for 8–10 minutes until softened.
3. Stir in the potatoes and courgettes, and cook for 5 minutes, stirring often. Add the tomatoes, hot stock and oregano and bring to the boil.
4. Reduce the heat to low, stir in the beans and simmer gently for 15 minutes or until the vegetables are tender. Stir in the spinach and parsley and cook for a further 5 minutes. Season to taste.
5. Ladle into bowls and drizzle with the chilli oil. Sprinkle with Parmesan and enjoy!

Or try this...
• Use any canned beans, e.g. borlotti, cannellini, haricot, flageolet.
• Add some dried soup pasta or broken spaghetti.
• Use canned tomatoes instead of fresh.

PER SERVING:

450 KCALS

19g PROTEIN

17g FAT

49g CARBS

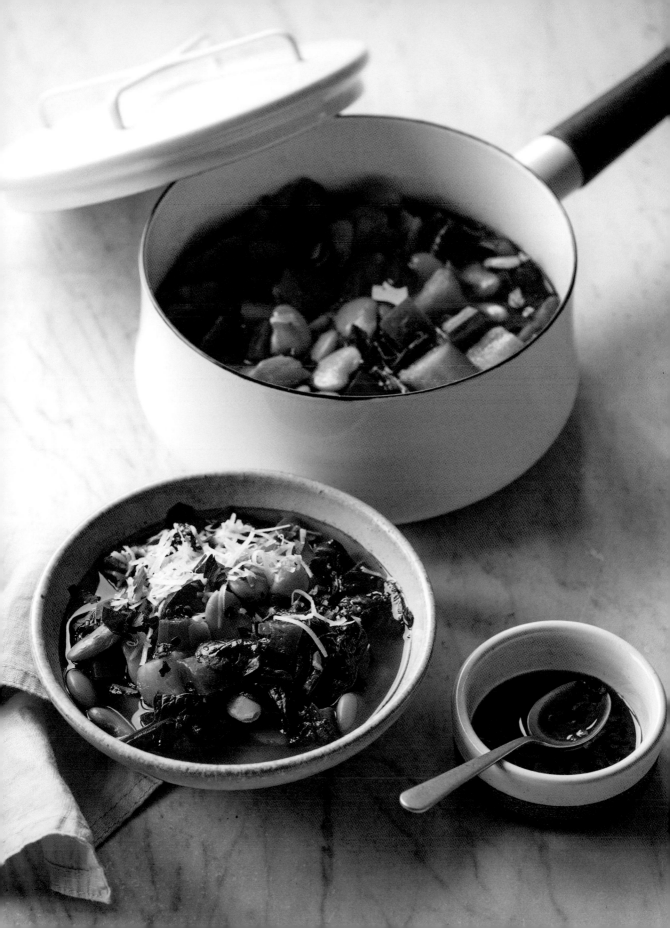

JAPANESE NOODLE SALAD JARS

Serves 2
Prep: 15 minutes
Cook: 10–15 minutes
Chill: several hours

100g (3½oz) soba noodles (dry
   weight)
150g (5oz/1 cup) frozen shelled
   edamame beans
1 red or yellow pepper, deseeded
   and diced
1 large carrot, shredded
4 spring onions, thinly sliced
a handful of rocket or watercress
salt and freshly ground black
   pepper

Peanut butter dressing:
2 tbsp peanut butter
2 tbsp light soy sauce
1 tbsp olive oil
2 tsp rice vinegar
juice of 1 lime
1 tsp runny honey
water for mixing
1 tsp black sesame seeds
a pinch of dried crushed red
   chilli flakes

For this salad, you'll need two wide-mouthed, tall Kilner or Mason jars with fitted glass lids, seals and clip tops. When you're assembling salad jars, always put the dressing in the bottom, then layer up the carbs, followed by firm vegetables, the protein, and, lastly, the salad leaves or greens. This stops them getting soggy and squashed. These jars make great packed lunches – so healthy and tasty!

1. Make the dressing: whisk together the peanut butter, soy sauce, oil, vinegar, lime juice and honey in a bowl until smooth. Whisk in a little cold water, just enough to give the dressing the consistency of cream. Stir in the sesame seeds and chilli flakes.
2. Cook the noodles according to the instructions on the packet. Rinse under cold running water, drain well and leave to cool.
3. Defrost the edamame beans according to the instructions on the packet.
4. Pour the dressing into the bottom of each glass jar and then divide the cooked noodles between the jars. Cover with the red or yellow pepper and carrot and then the edamame beans. Top with the spring onions and salad leaves and season with salt and pepper.
5. Cover the jars and chill in the fridge for several hours or overnight. When you're ready to eat, just tip everything out into 2 bowls and toss in the dressing.

Or try this...
• Add a layer of cold cooked chicken or cooked prawns.
• Stir some grated ginger or crushed garlic into the dressing.
• Substitute the chilli flakes with sweet chilli sauce.
• Use rice noodles or egg noodles.
• Add a layer of cucumber, sweetcorn or tomatoes.
• Vegans can use agave syrup instead of honey.

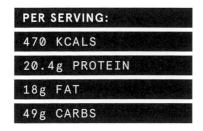

PER SERVING:
470 KCALS
20.4g PROTEIN
18g FAT
49g CARBS

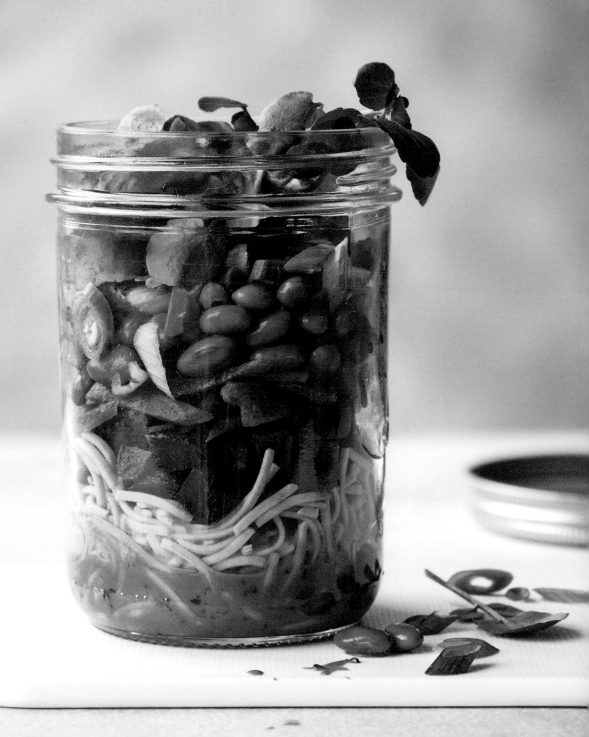

SPICY CHICKPEA BUDDHA BOWLS

Serves 2
Prep: 15 minutes
Cook: 30–35 minutes

1 x 400g (14oz) can chickpeas, rinsed and drained
½ tsp ground cumin seeds
½ tsp chilli powder
½ tsp smoked paprika
spray olive oil
1 small red onion, cut into wedges
1 red or yellow pepper, deseeded and cut into chunks
300g (10oz) pumpkin or butternut squash, peeled and cut into chunks
3 garlic cloves, unpeeled
200g (7oz) kale, trimmed
a handful of coriander or parsley, chopped
100g (3½oz/½ cup) couscous (dry weight)
180ml (6fl oz/¾ cup) boiling vegetable stock
balsamic vinegar, for drizzling
sea salt and freshly ground black pepper

PER SERVING:

395 KCALS

14.7g PROTEIN

5g FAT

32.4g CARBS

Packed with nutrients and flavour, this really is good food for your soul! Like many of the other lunches, you can make this in advance and portion it out into lunch boxes for the perfect midday meal. It's so versatile, so feel free to experiment and add whatever you've got handy in the fridge or kitchen cupboard.

1. Preheat the oven to 200ºC (180ºC fan/400ºF/gas 6).
2. Put the chickpeas in a bowl with the ground cumin seeds, chilli powder and smoked paprika. Add a pinch of sea salt, spray with oil and mix until the chickpeas are coated with the spices.
3. Spread out in a single layer on a baking tray and roast in the preheated oven, turning them once or twice, for 15–20 minutes, or until golden brown and slightly crisp. Leave to cool.
4. Put the onion, pepper and pumpkin or squash in a large roasting tin. Tuck the garlic cloves in between the vegetables and spray lightly with olive oil. Season with salt and pepper.
5. Roast in the preheated oven for 25–30 minutes, turning once or twice, until tender. Stir the kale into the roasted vegetables and return to the oven for 5 minutes. Squeeze the garlic out of the skins and stir into the vegetables with the chopped herbs.
6. Meanwhile, put the couscous in a heatproof bowl and pour over the hot stock. Cover and leave for 10–15 minutes until the couscous swells and absorbs the liquid. Fluff it up with a fork.
7. Divide the couscous, spiced chickpeas and roasted vegetables between 2 shallow serving bowls. Serve warm or cold, drizzled with balsamic vinegar.

Or try this...
• Use quinoa, brown rice or bulgur wheat instead of couscous.
• Drizzle with sweet chilli sauce or sriracha.
• Add some crumbled feta or goat's cheese.
• Try different veg – aubergine, cherry tomatoes or courgettes.

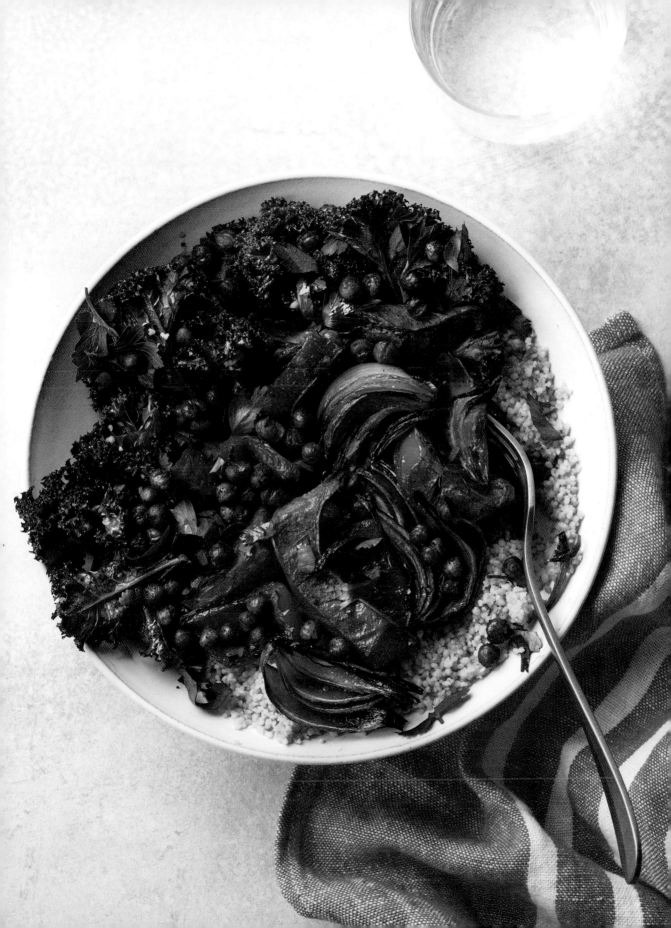

THAI LEFTOVER ROAST BEEF SALAD

Serves 2
Prep: 15 minutes

100g (3½oz) thin or vermicelli rice
    noodles (dry weight)
1 red pepper, deseeded and
    thinly sliced
1 large carrot, cut into
    matchsticks
½ cucumber, cut into
    matchsticks
4 spring onions, thinly sliced
a few crisp lettuce leaves, torn
a handful of coriander, chopped
200g (7oz) lean roast beef, all fat
    removed and meat sliced
30g (1oz/¼ cup) chopped roasted
    peanuts

Dressing:
1 red bird's eye chilli, shredded
2 garlic cloves, thinly sliced
2 tbsp Thai fish sauce (nam pla)
1 tbsp rice vinegar
juice of 1 lime
1 tsp caster sugar

This is such an amazing salad and it works on many levels. It has all my favourite Thai flavours, fills you up, and it's the perfect way to use up lovely rare leftover beef from the Sunday roast – it's great with chicken, too. If you're like me and crave a lot of heat, drizzle it with sweet chilli sauce or sriracha.

1. Cook the rice noodles according to the instructions on the packet. Drain well and cool.
2. Make the dressing: put all the ingredients in a bowl and whisk together until thoroughly combined.
3. Put the red pepper, carrot, cucumber, spring onions, lettuce and coriander in a large bowl and mix together gently.
4. Add the beef and rice noodles to the salad and toss in the dressing. Divide between 2 serving plates and sprinkle the peanuts over the top.

Or try this...
• Add 1 tsp sesame oil to the dressing.
• Instead of cold beef, use sliced grilled steaks or cooked prawns.

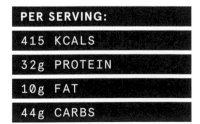

PER SERVING:
415 KCALS
32g PROTEIN
10g FAT
44g CARBS

MEXICAN BEAN SALAD LUNCH BOX

Serves 2
Prep: 15 minutes

1 x 400g (14oz) can red kidney
   beans, rinsed and drained
200g (7oz) cherry or baby plum
   tomatoes, quartered
½ red onion, thinly sliced
100g (3½oz) canned sweetcorn
   kernels in water, drained
a few crisp lettuce leaves, e.g.
   Little Gem, shredded
1 ripe avocado, peeled, stoned
   and cubed
a handful of coriander, chopped
100g (3½oz) feta cheese, diced

Dressing:
1 tbsp fruity green olive oil
1 tbsp sweet chilli sauce
1 tsp red or white wine vinegar
juice of 1 lime
1 garlic clove, crushed
a pinch of sugar

PER SERVING:
535 KCALS
14.7g PROTEIN
5g FAT
32.4g CARBS

This easy salad makes a delicious packed lunch or you can enjoy it at home. To make it more substantial and authentically Tex-Mex, fold or roll some wholemeal tortilla wraps around it, or you can use it as a filling for pitta pockets. Whatever rocks your boat.

1. Mix together the kidney beans, tomatoes, red onion, sweetcorn, lettuce, avocado and coriander in a bowl.
2. Make the dressing: blend all the ingredients together in a bowl or shake vigorously in a screw-top jar.
3. Pour the dressing over the kidney bean and sweetcorn mixture and toss gently. Add the feta and divide between 2 lunch-box containers. Cover securely with the lids and keep in the fridge or a cool place for up to 4–5 hours before eating.

Tip: You can, of course, eat the salad immediately for lunch or a light supper.

Or try this...
• Use lemon juice instead of lime.
• Add some shredded cooked chicken or prawns.
• Serve with a spoonful of tomato salsa or *pico de gallo*.
• Top with some guacamole and yoghurt.
• Add some diced red pepper.

SUSHI SALAD BOWL

Serves 2
Prep: 20 minutes
Cook: 10–15 minutes

75g (3oz/scant ½ cup) sushi rice
2 tbsp rice vinegar
1 tsp mirin
1 tsp black sesame seeds
1 tsp caster sugar
150g (5oz/1 cup) frozen shelled
   edamame beans
1 carrot, very thinly sliced
100g (3½oz) cherry tomatoes,
   halved or quartered
½ small cucumber, diced
2 spring onions, shredded
1 ripe avocado, peeled, stoned
   and cubed
a handful of salad leaves,
   shredded
150g (5oz) salmon fillet, cubed
sea salt
sprigs of coriander, chopped
nori strips, for sprinkling

Wasabi dressing:
2 tbsp light soy sauce
1 tbsp rice vinegar
juice of ½ lime
1 tsp wasabi
a pinch of sugar

PER SERVING:

550 KCALS
32g PROTEIN
24g FAT
40.8g CARBS

Sushi fans will love this healthy salad. It's very important to buy really good-quality fresh salmon, preferably sashimi grade for the best results. However, if you like Japanese umami flavours but are squeamish about eating raw salmon why not cheat and use sliced smoked salmon instead?

1. Cook the rice according to the instructions on the packet – it will take 10–15 minutes until it's tender and all (or most) of the water has been absorbed.
2. Heat the rice vinegar, mirin, sesame seeds and sugar in a small saucepan over a low heat, stirring to dissolve the sugar. Mix gently into the rice, then cover the pan and leave for 10 minutes, or until the rice is at room temperature.
3. Meanwhile, defrost the edamame beans according to the instructions on the packet.
4. Make the wasabi dressing: whisk all the ingredients in a bowl until well blended.
5. Put the edamame beans, carrot, tomatoes, cucumber, spring onions, avocado and salad leaves in a bowl and toss lightly in the dressing. Check the seasoning, adding salt if wished.
6. Divide the rice between 2 shallow serving bowls. Pile the salad on top with the salmon cubes. Sprinkle with the coriander and nori strips and serve.

Tip: Sushi rice, mirin, nori and wasabi are available in most supermarkets as well as delis.

Or try this...
- Sprinkle with white sesame seeds.
- Add some Japanese pickled ginger.
- Vary the salad: add some radishes or red pepper.

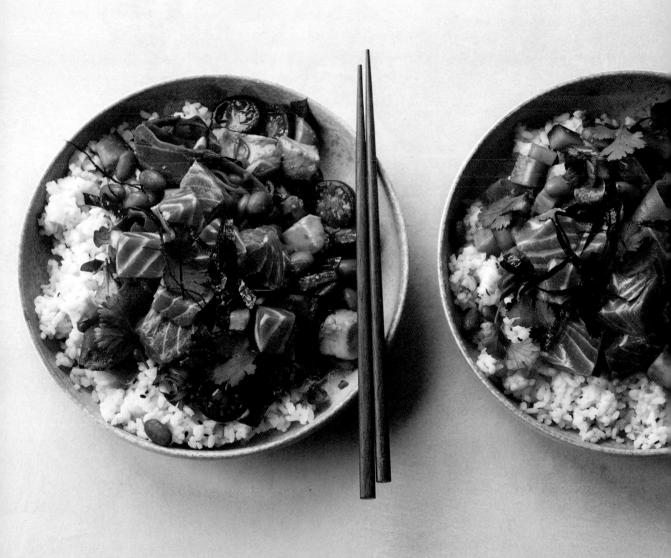

STEAK AND RICE NOODLE RAMEN

Serves 2
Prep: 15 minutes
Cook: 15 minutes

250g (9oz) ramen noodles (dry
   weight)
1 tbsp olive oil, plus extra for
   brushing
300g (10oz) shiitake mushrooms,
   sliced
1 large carrot, cut into
   matchsticks
2 garlic cloves, thinly sliced
2.5cm (1in) piece fresh root
   ginger, peeled and diced
1 red chilli, deseeded and
   shredded
1 litre (33fl oz/generous 4 cups)
   hot beef stock
2 tbsp miso paste
2 tbsp soy sauce
200g (7oz) pak choi, trimmed
   and sliced
100g (3½oz) mangetout, trimmed
1 bunch of spring onions,
   shredded
juice of 1 lime
400g (14oz) lean rump or sirloin
   steak, all visible fat removed
chopped coriander, to garnish

PER SERVING:
500 KCALS
37.5g PROTEIN
24g FAT
31.6g CARBS

This Japanese meal-in-a-bowl is real comfort food and surprisingly quick and easy to make. It's a great source of protein, vitamins and minerals, and very uplifting on a cold day. Keep a tub of miso paste in your fridge – it will stay fresh for up to a month. When you feel like a hot drink or a snack, just stir a spoonful into a mug of hot beef, chicken or vegetable stock.

1. Cook the noodles according to the instructions on the packet. Drain well.
2. Meanwhile, heat the oil in a large saucepan over a medium heat. Add the mushrooms and carrot and cook, stirring occasionally, for 5 minutes, or until the carrot is just tender. Stir in the garlic, ginger and chilli, and cook for 1 minute.
3. Reduce the heat and add the stock, miso paste and soy sauce. Simmer for 5 minutes before adding the pak choi, mangetout and spring onions. Cook gently for 2–3 minutes, until the mangetout is just tender but still crisp and the pak choi starts to wilt. Add the lime juice.
4. Meanwhile, grill the steak in a lightly oiled griddle pan over a high heat for 3–5 minutes until browned on both sides and cooked to your liking. Remove and cut into thin strips.
5. Divide the noodles between 2 shallow bowls and ladle the hot soup over them. Top with the steak, then sprinkle with coriander and serve.

Tip: You can use white or brown miso paste – the brown has a more distinctive and earthy taste.

Or try this...
• Add some shredded Chinese cabbage at the end.
• Substitute tamari for the soy sauce.

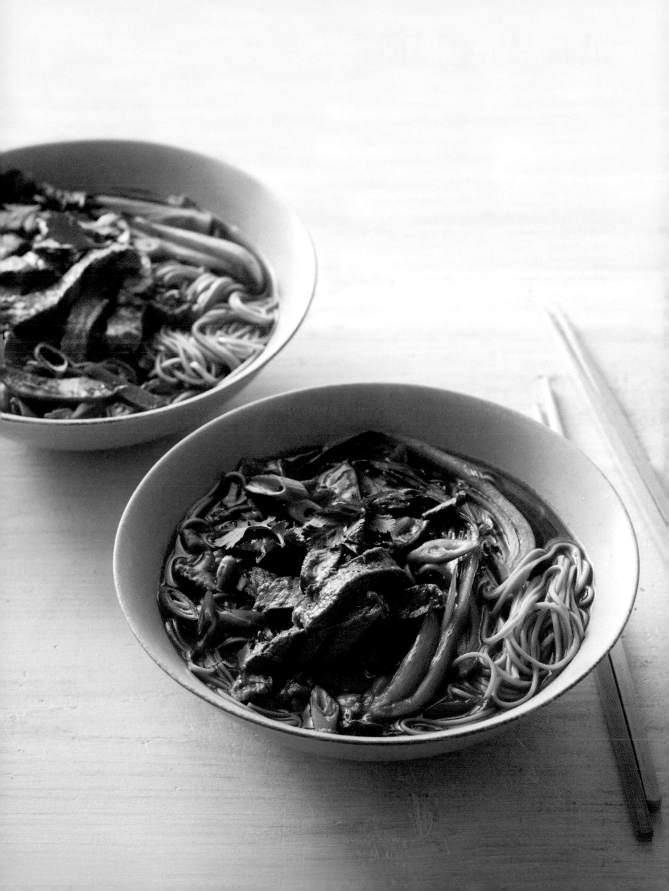

WARM LENTIL SALAD

Serves 2
Prep: 15 minutes
Cook: 20 minutes

200g (7oz/1 cup) Puy or green
   lentils (dry weight)
2 tbsp olive oil
1 onion, finely chopped
1 large carrot, finely diced
2 celery sticks, diced
2 garlic cloves, crushed
200g (7oz) baby plum tomatoes,
   halved
100g (3½oz) baby spinach leaves
juice of 1 lemon
a few drops of balsamic vinegar
a handful of dill, chopped
100g (3½oz) smoked salmon,
   thinly sliced
4 tbsp 0% fat Greek yoghurt
1 lemon, quartered
salt and freshly ground black
   pepper

PER SERVING:
495 KCALS
22g PROTEIN
21g FAT
26.6g CARBS

Lentils are among the healthiest foods you can eat, especially if you're looking for plant protein. For salads, you need to use the small green, brown or black lentils which keep their shape when they're cooked. Avoid the red ones that go soft and mushy – they are better for making soups and dhal.

1. Put the lentils in a saucepan and cover with cold water. Bring to the boil, then reduce the heat and simmer gently for 15–20 minutes, or until they are tender but still have a little bite. Drain and refresh under cold running water.

2. Meanwhile, heat the oil in a large frying pan over a low heat. Add the onion, carrot, celery and garlic and cook for 8–10 minutes, or until they are really tender.

3. Add the tomatoes and cooked lentils and cook for 5 minutes, stirring occasionally. If the lentils start to stick, add a little water. Stir in the baby spinach leaves and cook for 2 minutes until they wilt. Add the lemon juice, balsamic vinegar and most of the dill. Season to taste with salt and pepper. Remove from the heat and set aside for 10 minutes.

4. Divide the lukewarm lentils between 2 serving plates with the smoked salmon and yoghurt. Sprinkle the yoghurt with the remaining dill and serve with lemon quarters for squeezing.

Tip: This looks great if you roll up the smoked salmon slices.

Or try this...
• Instead of salmon, serve with sliced mozzarella, burrata, crumbled feta or some grilled halloumi.
• Use basil or mint instead of dill.
• Stir some mustardy vinaigrette dressing into the cooked lentils.

GREEK-STYLE VEGGIE PITTA POCKETS

Serves 2
Prep: 15 minutes
Cook: 15 minutes

1 large aubergine, thickly sliced
1 red pepper, deseeded and
    sliced
1 red onion, cut into rounds
2 tbsp olive oil
1 tsp za'atar
1 tsp dried oregano
2 large wholemeal pitta breads
a handful of crisp lettuce, e.g.
    Cos or Little Gem, shredded
100g (3½oz) feta cheese, cubed
salt and freshly ground black
    pepper
lemon wedges, for squeezing

Tzatziki:
100g (3½oz/scant ½ cup) 0% fat
    Greek yoghurt
1 tsp fruity olive oil
¼ cucumber, diced
1–2 garlic cloves, crushed
a small handful of mint or dill,
    finely chopped
grated zest and juice of ½ lemon

PER SERVING:

540 KCALS

23.8g PROTEIN

35g FAT

44g CARBS

These fabulous warm pitta breads are filled with griddled vegetables, feta and tzatziki – that's as Greek as it gets. Vegans can use dairy-free yoghurt and cashew cheese or griddled tofu in the filling.

1. Make the tzatziki: mix all the ingredients together in a bowl. Season to taste with salt and pepper.
2. Brush the aubergine, red pepper and onion with olive oil on both sides. Sprinkle with the za'atar and oregano, and season with salt and pepper.
3. Place a large ridged griddle pan over a medium to high heat and cook the oiled vegetables in batches, a few at a time, for 2–3 minutes on each side, or until charred and golden brown. Drain on kitchen paper and keep warm.
4. Warm the pitta breads on the griddle pan then split them open down one side. Fill with the shredded lettuce, griddled vegetables and feta and drizzle with tzatziki. Eat immediately while they are warm, with some lemon wedges for squeezing.

Tip: if you wrap some kitchen foil or baking parchment round the pitta breads, it makes them easier to hold while you're eating them.

Or try this...
• Use hummus instead of tzatziki.
• Drizzle with hot sauce or add a dash of harissa.
• Add some grilled halloumi or tofu.
• Use wholemeal wraps or soft flatbreads instead of pitta.

DINNERS

CHICKEN PICCATA

Serves 2
Prep: 10 minutes
Cook: 15 minutes

100g (3½oz/generous ½ cup)
   wholegrain brown rice
a good pinch of paprika
a pinch of dried crushed red chilli
   flakes
2 x 150g (5oz) skinned and boned
   chicken breasts
plain or almond flour, for dusting
2 tbsp olive oil
2 tbsp capers
2 garlic cloves, crushed
grated zest and juice of 1 lemon
200ml (7fl oz/scant 1 cup) hot
   chicken stock
1 small lemon, sliced
a handful of parsley, chopped
salt and freshly ground black
   pepper
green vegetables, e.g. beans or
   broccoli, to serve

PER SERVING:

510 KCALS

40g PROTEIN

18.5g FAT

37.5g CARBS

This is the perfect supper when you're in a hurry or feeling done in after a day's work. There aren't many ingredients, it's quick and easy to make, it's cooked in one pan *and* it tastes awesome. What's not to like?

1. Cook the rice according to the instructions on the packet. Fluff up with a fork, dust with the paprika and stir in the chilli flakes.
2. Meanwhile, slice each chicken breast through the middle lengthways, leaving a little bit uncut at the end, and open it up like a book. Place between 2 sheets of baking parchment or cling film and flatten with a rolling pin or mallet. Lightly dust the chicken on both sides with flour.
3. Heat the oil in a large frying pan over a medium heat. Add the chicken and fry for 4 minutes on each side or until cooked through and golden brown. Remove from the pan and set aside.
4. Add the capers and garlic to the pan and cook for 1 minute. Add the lemon zest and juice and the hot stock and let it bubble away for 5 minutes, until the sauce reduces and thickens. Return the cooked chicken to the pan and stir in the sliced lemon and parsley. Season to taste with salt and pepper.
5. Serve the rice with the chicken in the lemony sauce, and some green vegetables.

Or you can try...
• Serve with pasta or noodles instead of rice.
• If you're cutting down on carbs, this tastes great with cauliflower 'rice' or courgetti 'noodles'.
• Use turkey escalopes instead of chicken.
• Add some crème fraîche or coconut cream to the sauce.

STEAK TAGLIATA

Serves 2
Prep: 15 minutes
Cook: 30–35 minutes

300g (10oz) new potatoes,
  halved or quartered
2 tbsp olive oil, plus extra for
  brushing
2–3 garlic cloves, crushed
leaves stripped from 2 rosemary
  sprigs
100g (3½oz) rocket
200g (7oz) baby plum or cherry
  tomatoes, halved
2 x 150g (5oz) lean sirloin steaks,
  all visible fat removed
25g (1oz) Parmesan cheese,
  shaved with a potato peeler
salt and freshly ground black
  pepper

Dressing:
1 tbsp fruity olive oil
juice of ½ lemon
1 tbsp balsamic vinegar
1 tsp honey mustard

PER SERVING:
605 KCALS
46g PROTEIN
33.7g FAT
27g CARBS

Most of us like a nice juicy steak for supper, and this Italian way of serving it with crispy, garlicky potatoes is delicious. Make sure you use really lean sirloin steaks and cut off any visible fat before cooking them.

1. Preheat the oven to 180ºC (160ºC fan/350ºF/gas 4).
2. Toss the new potatoes in a bowl with the olive oil, garlic and rosemary. Season with salt and pepper. Tip into a roasting tin and roast in the preheated oven for 30–35 minutes, or until tender, golden brown and crispy.
3. Meanwhile, make the dressing: whisk all the ingredients together. Gently toss the rocket and tomatoes in a bowl with the dressing.
4. Lightly brush the steaks with oil and season with plenty of salt and pepper. Set a heavy frying pan over a high heat and when it's smoking hot add the steaks. Sear for 2–3 minutes each side for rare to medium-rare – longer if you like them well done. Remove from the pan and leave to rest on a chopping board.
5. Cut the warm steaks into slices and arrange on 2 serving plates with the crispy new potatoes and rocket salad. Sprinkle the Parmesan shavings over the salad and serve immediately.

Tip: Use a ridged griddle pan if you like your steak slightly charred and attractively striped.

Or try this...
• Use a packet of ready-washed mixed rocket, watercress and spinach.
• Fry leftover cooked new potatoes in some oil with garlic and herbs in a pan.

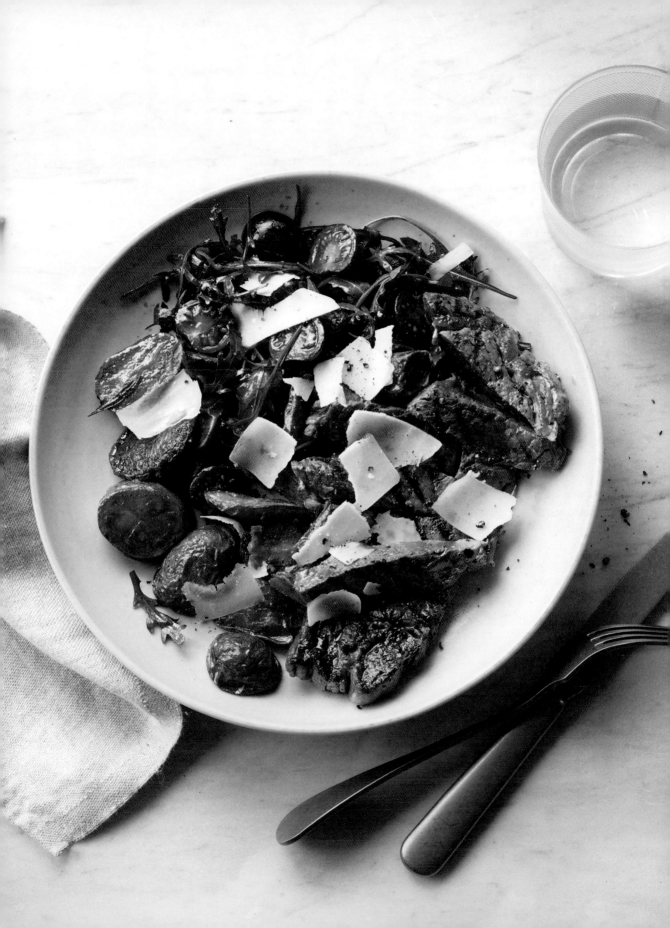

CHICKEN MILANESE

Serves 2
Prep: 25 minutes
Cook: 15 minutes

2 x 150g (5oz) skinned and boned
   chicken breasts
plain flour, for dusting
1 medium free-range egg,
   beaten
45g (1½oz/½ cup) dried
   breadcrumbs
25g (1oz/¼ cup) grated
   Parmesan cheese
3 tbsp light olive oil
sea salt and freshly ground black
   pepper

Orange and fennel salad:
1 large fennel bulb, trimmed
2 juicy oranges
10 black olives
seeds of 1 pomegranate
fruity green olive oil, for drizzling
crushed sea salt crystals

PER SERVING:

660 KCALS

46g PROTEIN

34g FAT

35g CARBS

This is as good as it gets: succulent fried chicken escalopes served with a crisp, tangy Sicilian salad of fennel, orange and juicy black olives. The fennel has a wonderful aniseedy flavour and is great for your digestive system. I like to cook double the amount of chicken breasts and eat the leftover ones cold the next day.

1. Make the salad: thinly slice the fennel and place in a bowl. Chop the small stalks and feathery fronds and set aside.
2. Cut the tops and bases off each orange and then remove the outer peel and white pith with a sharp knife. Cut each orange horizontally into slices and add to the fennel with any juice.
3. Scatter with the olives, pomegranate seeds and reserved fennel stalks and fronds, and gently mix everything together. Drizzle with olive oil and some crushed sea salt crystals. Set aside while you prepare and cook the chicken.
4. Cut each chicken breast in half horizontally. Place between 2 sheets of greaseproof paper or cling film and flatten with a mallet or a rolling pin until 5mm (¼in) thick.
5. Lightly dust each chicken breast with flour on both sides and then dip into the beaten egg. Mix the breadcrumbs and grated Parmesan on a plate and use to coat the chicken on both sides.
6. Heat the oil in a large frying pan set over a medium to high heat. When it's really hot, add the chicken breasts, in batches, and sauté for 3–4 minutes on each side until they are cooked right through and golden brown and crisp. Remove and drain on kitchen paper. Serve immediately with the salad.

Or try this...
• Use turkey or veal escalopes instead of chicken.
• Use blood oranges (ruby red oranges or sanguinelli). The colour is sensational.

GREEK-STYLE LAMB BURGERS

Serves 2
Prep: 15 minutes
Chill: 15 minutes
Cook: 8–10 minutes

300g (10oz/scant 1½ cups)
  extra-lean minced lamb
2 garlic cloves, crushed
a few sprigs of mint, leaves finely
  chopped
¼ tsp ground cumin
¼ tsp ground cinnamon
a pinch of fennel seeds
100g (3½oz/generous ½ cup)
  wholegrain brown rice
1 tbsp light olive oil
salt and freshly ground black
  pepper
salad or vegetables, to serve

Tahini sauce:
1 garlic clove, crushed
½ tsp sea salt flakes
2 tbsp tahini
juice of ½ lemon
2 spring onions, thinly sliced
100g (3½oz/scant ½ cup) 0% fat
  Greek yoghurt
a few sprigs of mint, chopped

PER SERVING:
585 KCALS
49g PROTEIN
29g FAT
41g CARBS

These subtly spiced burgers with nutty brown rice make a filling supper. You can even prepare the burgers the day before and keep them in the fridge overnight before cooking. And they taste smoky and even better when they're cooked over glowing hot coals on the barbie on a summer's day.

1. Mix together the lamb, garlic, mint, spices and seeds in a bowl. Season with salt and pepper, then shape into 4 burgers. Chill in the fridge for at least 15 minutes to firm them up.
2. Meanwhile, make the tahini sauce: crush the garlic and salt and mix in a bowl with the tahini and lemon juice. Add the spring onions, yoghurt and chopped mint and stir well.
3. Cook the rice according to the instructions on the packet.
4. Lightly brush a ridged griddle pan or frying pan with the oil and set over a medium heat. When it's hot, cook the burgers for 4–5 minutes each side, depending on how well cooked you like them. The outer crust should be well browned and crisp. Drain briefly on kitchen paper.
5. Serve the burgers, drizzled with the tahini sauce, with the brown rice and some salad or griddled vegetables.

Tip: If you can't find any extra-lean minced lamb, buy some really lean fillet or leg steaks and mince the meat yourself or blitz it in a food processor.

Or try this...
• Swirl some hot harissa paste into the tahini sauce.
• Serve with tzatziki or hummus.
• Serve the burgers in toasted buns, pittas or flatbreads.
• Use dried oregano or chopped fresh coriander instead of mint.
• Use minced beef or chicken.

CAULI 'STEAKS' WITH MARINARA SAUCE

Serves 2
Prep: 20 minutes
Cook: 25 minutes

1 small cauliflower, stalk trimmed
    and leaves discarded
1 tbsp olive oil, plus extra for
    brushing
2 garlic cloves, crushed
leaves from 2 thyme sprigs
a pinch of dried red chilli flakes
2 tbsp grated Parmesan cheese
100g (3½oz/generous ½ cup)
    quinoa (dry weight)
salt and freshly ground black
    pepper

Marinara sauce:
1 tbsp olive oil
1 small red onion, diced
1 garlic clove, crushed
1 red chilli, deseeded and diced
400g (14oz) tomatoes, chopped
1 tbsp tomato paste
a pinch of sugar
a handful of fresh basil leaves
1 tsp balsamic vinegar
1 x 400g (14oz) can chickpeas,
    rinsed and drained

PER SERVING:
625 KCALS
22.3g PROTEIN
16.8g FAT
60g CARBS

Cauliflower 'steaks' are the new faux meat. They are a good source of plant protein and a delicious and economical vegetarian alternative to the real thing. In this tasty supper, the chickpeas and quinoa provide additional protein and dietary fibre.

1. Preheat the oven to 200ºC (180ºC fan/400ºF/gas 6).
2. Slice the cauliflower through the stem into 4 thick 'steaks'. Heat the oil in a large frying pan over a high heat. Add the cauliflower steaks to the pan, two at a time, and cook for 2 minutes on each side, until starting to colour.
3. Lightly brush a large baking sheet with oil. Add the cauliflower and sprinkle with the garlic, thyme, chilli flakes and some salt and pepper. Roast in the preheated oven for 15 minutes, then sprinkle with the Parmesan. Roast for another 5 minutes, or until tender, golden brown and slightly charred around the edges.
4. Cook the quinoa according to the instructions on the packet.
5. While the quinoa is cooking, make the sauce: add the oil to the pan in which the cauliflower was cooked and reduce the heat to medium. Add the onion, garlic and chilli and cook, stirring occasionally, for 6–8 minutes, or until softened. Stir in the tomatoes, tomato paste, sugar and basil and cook for 5 minutes until thickened. Add the balsamic and season to taste.
6. Blitz three-quarters of the mixture in a blender or food processor until smooth – alternatively, crush the tomatoes with a wooden spoon for a coarser sauce. Return the blitzed sauce to the pan and stir in the chickpeas. Heat through gently.
7. Serve the cauliflower at once with the sauce and quinoa.

Or try this...
• Drizzle the cauliflower with some pesto.
• Use canned chopped tomatoes instead of fresh.
• Add some diced black olives to the sauce.

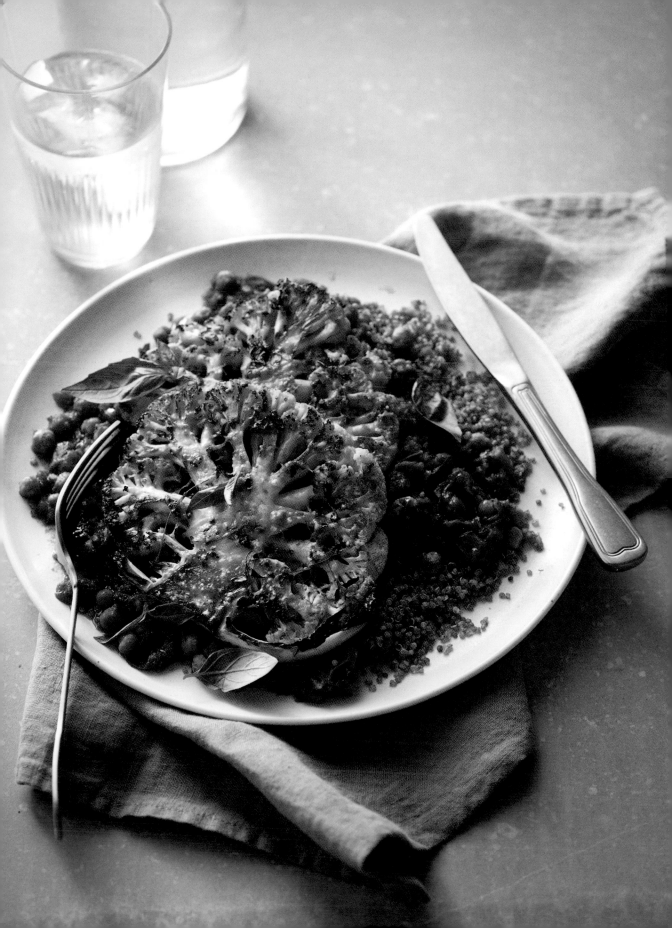

FLASH-IN-THE-PAN FISH FILLETS

Serves 2
Prep: 10 minutes
Cook: 20 minutes

400g (14oz) new potatoes, halved or cut into chunks
2 tbsp olive oil
2 red or yellow peppers, deseeded and sliced
2 garlic cloves, crushed
300g (10oz) ripe tomatoes, chopped
8 black olives, stoned and chopped
120ml (4fl oz/½ cup) hot fish or vegetable stock
2 x 150g (5oz) skinned sea bass fillets
a handful of flat-leaf parsley, chopped
salt and freshly ground black pepper
green vegetables e.g. beans or broccoli, to serve

PER SERVING:
590 KCALS
34g PROTEIN
31.7g FAT
40g CARBS

Variations on this dish are eaten all around the Mediterranean, especially in Spain, southern Italy and Greece. I usually use sea bass but any white fish fillets work well. It will still be really tasty.

1. Cook the potatoes in a pan of boiling salted water for 15 minutes, or until tender. Drain well and keep warm.
2. Meanwhile, heat the oil in a large frying pan over a medium heat. Add the peppers and cook, stirring occasionally, for 5 minutes, or until tender. Add the garlic and cook for 1 minute.
3. Stir in the tomatoes, olives and stock and cook for 2–3 minutes. Add the fish fillets, then cover the pan and cook for 8 minutes, or until they are cooked right through and opaque. Check the pan once or twice while they're cooking – if the sauce is sticking or getting too thick, add some more stock or water. Stir in the parsley and season to taste with salt and pepper.
4. Divide between 2 serving plates. Serve with the new potatoes and some green vegetables.

Or try this...
• You can use peeled regular potatoes cut into chunks instead of new potatoes.
• Use cod, haddock, plaice or lemon sole fillets.
• Use canned instead of fresh tomatoes.
• Add some onion, courgette or spinach to the sauce.

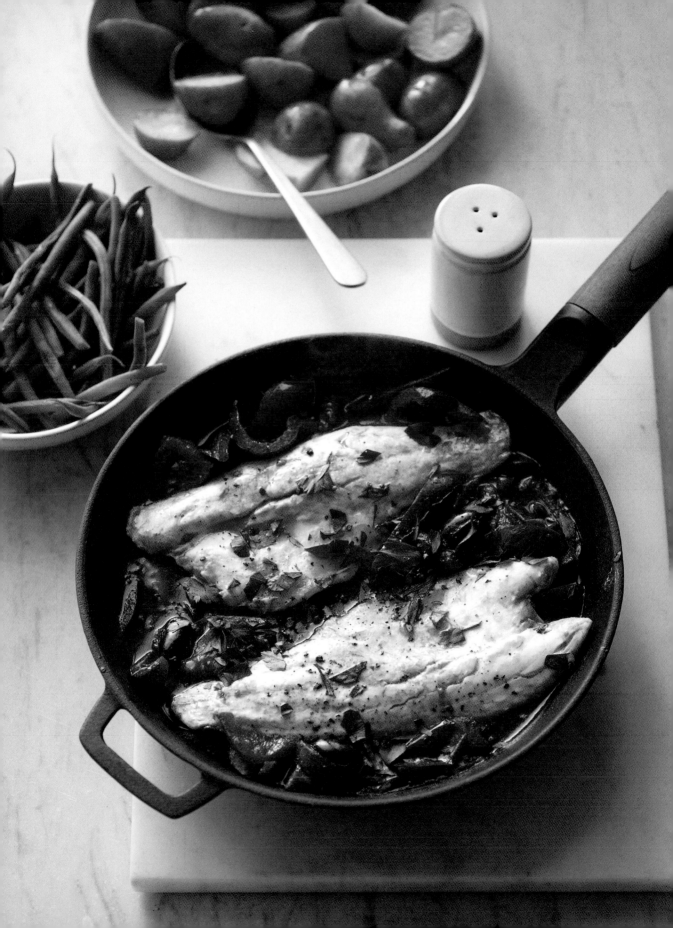

PIRI PIRI CHICKEN WITH FRUITY COLESLAW

Serves 2
Prep: 20 minutes
Cook: 25–35 minutes

2 medium sweet potatoes
  (approx. 200g/7oz each)
spray olive oil
2 tsp paprika
1 tsp garlic powder
½ tsp cayenne
a few sprigs of rosemary and
  thyme
1 tbsp sriracha (or hot sauce)
grated zest and juice of ½ lemon
2 garlic cloves, crushed
2 x 125g (4 ½oz) skinned and
  boned chicken breasts
salt and black pepper

Fruity coleslaw:
100g (3½oz) white cabbage,
  thinly shredded
2 carrots, grated
½ red onion, grated
1 red apple, cored and diced
2 tbsp chopped walnuts
2 tsp mixed seeds
a handful of flat-leaf parsley
2 tbsp light mayonnaise
2 tbsp 0% fat Greek yoghurt
juice of ½ small lemon

PER SERVING:
595 KCALS
41g PROTEIN
18g FAT
62g CARBS

This delicious dinner for two is nearly as quick as ordering a take-away. I love cooking from scratch at home. It's much healthier, lower in calories and there are no surprises – I know exactly what's in it. If you're in a hurry, you could cheat and use supermarket coleslaw but it won't be half as good.

1. Preheat the oven to 200ºC (180ºC fan/400ºF/gas mark 6).
2. Cut the sweet potatoes into wedges. Spray lightly with oil and sprinkle with the paprika, garlic powder, cayenne and black pepper. Place in a roasting tin and sprinkle the herbs and some sea salt over the top. Bake in the preheated oven for 25–30 minutes, or until tender and golden brown.
3. Meanwhile, make the coleslaw: mix all the ingredients together in a bowl, and season to taste with salt and pepper.
4. In another bowl, mix the sriracha, lemon zest, juice and garlic. Add the chicken breasts and coat them all over in the mixture.
5. Lightly spray a griddle pan or non-stick frying pan with oil and cook the chicken breasts over a medium heat for 15 minutes, turning them over halfway through, or until golden brown and cooked right through.
6. Serve immediately with the coleslaw and spicy sweet potato wedges.

Tip: Make the coleslaw the day before and keep it in a sealed container in the fridge.

Or try this...
• Use red cabbage or some kale instead of white.
• Use spring onions in the coleslaw.
• Add some thinly sliced fennel or celery to the slaw.

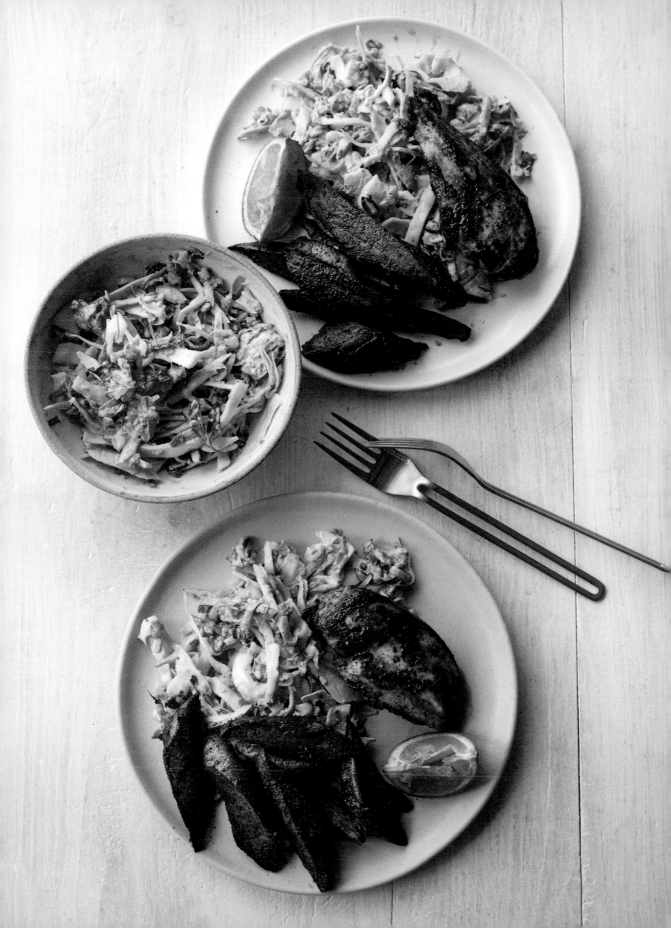

JAPANESE TOFU AND BLACK BEAN RICE BOWL

Serves 2
Prep: 10 minutes
Cook: 15–20 minutes

100g (3½oz/scant ½ cup)
    wholegrain brown rice
225g (8oz) smoked tofu
spray olive oil
½ tsp smoked paprika
100g (3½oz) tenderstem broccoli
1 x 400g (14oz) can black beans,
    rinsed and drained
¼ cucumber, diced or cut into
    matchsticks
1 ripe small avocado, peeled,
    stoned and cubed
a handful of coriander, chopped
1 tsp black or white sesame seeds
1 sheet ready-toasted sushi nori,
    cut into thin shreds
salt and freshly ground black
    pepper

Dressing:
1 tbsp rice vinegar
2 tsp soy sauce
1 tsp toasted sesame oil
1 tsp mirin

I always have brown rice in preference to white. It's much healthier as it's a whole grain with the fibrous bran intact and it's choc-a-bloc with protein, fibre, B vitamins and magnesium. Plus, I like its nutty taste and slightly crunchy texture. If you're like me, and love Japanese food, this is a great way to eat it.

1. Preheat the oven to 220ºC (200ºC fan/425ºF/gas 7).
2. Cook the brown rice according to the instructions on the packet. Fluff up with a fork and keep warm.
3. Blot the tofu with kitchen paper and cut into cubes. Lightly spray with oil and dust with the smoked paprika. Season with salt and pepper and place on a baking tray. Bake in the preheated oven for 15 minutes, or until golden and crisp.
4. Meanwhile, cut the broccoli stems in half lengthways and cook in boiling water for 2 minutes, or until they are just tender but still retain their 'bite'. Drain well.
5. Make the dressing: mix all the ingredients together in a small jug.
6. Mix the cooked rice with the broccoli and black beans, and toss gently in the dressing. Divide between 2 shallow serving bowls and arrange the cucumber, avocado and tofu on top. Sprinkle with the coriander, sesame seeds and nori, and serve immediately.

Or try this...
- Use small broccoli florets instead of tenderstem broccoli.
- Use canned red kidney beans or edamame beans.
- Instead of cucumber, use some carrot matchsticks or sliced radishes.
- Flavour the dressing with some Japanese pickled ginger.

PER SERVING:
610 KCALS
31g PROTEIN
21g FAT
59g CARBS

STORE-CUPBOARD SPAGHETTI WITH SARDINES

Serves 2
Prep: 5 minutes
Cook: 15–20 minutes

3 tbsp extra virgin olive oil
50g (2oz/1 cup) fresh
    breadcrumbs
1 small onion, diced
2 garlic cloves, crushed
1 juicy lemon
a few crushed dried red chilli
    flakes
2 x 120g (4oz) cans sardines in
    ollve oil, drained
4 tbsp capers, rinsed
200g (7oz) gluten-free spaghetti
    (dry weight)
a handful of flat-leaf parsley,
    chopped
sea salt and freshly ground black
    pepper

PER SERVING:

660 KCALS

28.6g PROTEIN

37g FAT

64.5g CARBS

When you're training hard as well as working and looking after your family and home, there's not much time to shop. Don't worry! Help is at hand. This supper is made with ingredients we all keep in our store cupboards. I use gluten-free pasta because it fills me up without leaving me feeling bloated.

1. Heat 2 tablespoons of the olive oil in a frying pan over a low to medium heat, add the breadcrumbs and fry, stirring occasionally, for 3–4 minutes, or until crisp and golden brown. Remove from the pan and drain on kitchen paper.
2. Add the remaining oil to the pan (or use a fresh pan, if you like) and cook the onion and garlic for 6–8 minutes until softened and golden. Peel a long strip of lemon rind and add to the pan with the chilli flakes, sardines and capers. Reduce the heat to very low and cook gently for 5 minutes, pressing down on the sardines to break them up. Remove the lemon zest.
3. Cook the spaghetti according to the instructions on the packet.
4. Drain the spaghetti, reserving the cooking water. Add to the sardine mixture, together with the juice of the lemon and the parsley. Stir in some of the reserved cooking water, a little at a time, until the oil and lemon juice combine with the starchy water to make a smooth sauce. Season to taste.
5. Divide between 2 serving plates and sprinkle with the crispy fried breadcrumbs.

Tip: Use good-quality canned sardines and add some of the drained oil to the sauce.

Or try this...
• Sprinkle with grated lemon zest or toasted pine nuts.
• Use chopped chives or dill instead or parsley.
• Add some courgettes, peas or green beans.

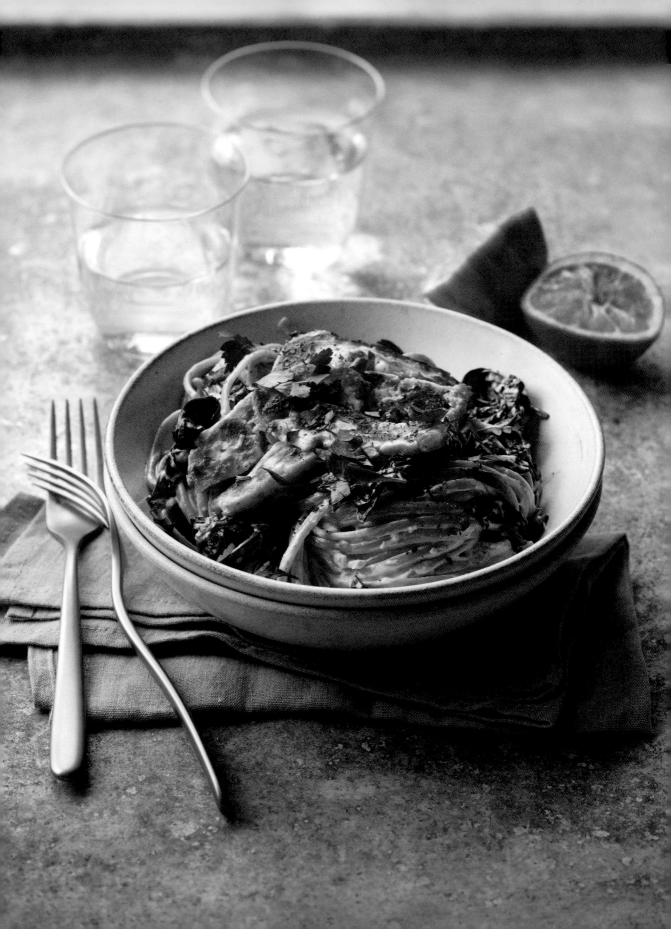

LEMONY LINGUINE
WITH CRISPY HALLOUMI

Serves 2
Prep: 5 minutes
Cook: 10 minutes

1 free-range egg yolk
120ml (4fl oz/½ cup) half-fat
   crème fraîche
25g (1oz/¼ cup) grated
   Parmesan cheese
grated zest and juice of 1 large
   juicy lemon
250g (9oz) gluten-free linguine
   (dry weight)
100g (3½oz) halloumi, thinly
   sliced
1 tbsp fruity green olive oil
200g (7oz) baby spinach leaves
salt and freshly ground black
   pepper
a few sprigs of flat-leaf parsley,
   finely chopped, to serve

PER SERVING:

620 KCALS

24.3g PROTEIN

28g FAT

48g CARBS

Even if you're a committed meat and fish eater,
you will love this vegetarian supper of pasta in a
creamy lemon and spinach sauce topped with
crispy halloumi. To keep the calories and fat
content low, I use half-fat crème fraîche.

1. Beat the egg yolk, crème fraîche, grated Parmesan, and the
   lemon zest and juice together in a bowl until well combined.
2. Cook the pasta in a large saucepan of salted boiling water
   according to the instructions on the packet.
3. Meanwhile, dry-fry the halloumi in a non-stick frying pan over
   a medium heat for 1–2 minutes on each side until any liquid
   has been released and evaporated and the halloumi is golden
   brown and crispy on the outside and softened inside. Remove
   from the pan and keep warm.
4. Drain the pasta, reserving a little of the cooking liquid, and
   return to the warm pan. Off the heat, stir in the olive oil and
   spinach leaves – they will wilt and turn bright green. Gently stir
   in the lemon mixture to coat all the strands of pasta. Season to
   taste with salt and pepper. If the sauce is too thick for your liking,
   add a little of the pasta cooking liquid to thin it.
5. Divide between 2 shallow serving bowls and top with the crispy
   halloumi. Sprinkle with the parsley and serve immediately.

Tip: Dry-fry the halloumi at the last moment, just before serving.
As it cools down, it will lose its crispness and the texture will
become more rubbery.

Or try this...
• Substitute 0% fat Greek yoghurt for the crème fraîche and save
   on calories and fat grams.
• Sprinkle with chopped mint or torn basil leaves.
• Top with more grated Parmesan.

VEGAN TACOS

Serves 2
Prep: 15 minutes
Cook: 15–20 minutes

1 tbsp olive oil
1 red onion, finely chopped
2 garlic cloves, crushed
1 tsp chilli powder
½ tsp smoked paprika
2 ripe tomatoes, chopped
1 x 400g (14oz) can chickpeas,
   rinsed and drained
50g (2oz/generous ¼ cup)
   canned sweetcorn kernels,
   drained
a handful of coriander, chopped
200g (7oz) firm tofu, cubed
85g (3oz/½ cup) wholegrain
   brown rice
4 hard taco shells
salt and freshly ground black
   pepper
fresh tomato salsa, dairy-free
   yoghurt and lime wedges,
   to serve

PER SERVING:

660 KCALS
23g PROTEIN
22.8g FAT
65g CARBS

These crisp tacos, with their spicy filling of chickpeas and crispy tofu are very healthy and nutritious. And they pack quite a plant protein punch. You don't have to use taco shells – warm some wholewheat tortillas in a griddle pan and then fold or roll them around the filling if you prefer.

1. Heat some of the oil in a large frying pan set over a low to medium heat. Add the onion and garlic and cook, stirring occasionally, for 6–8 minutes until tender. Stir in the chilli powder and paprika and cook for 1 minute. Reduce the heat to low and add the tomatoes, chickpeas and sweetcorn and cook for 5 minutes, or until reduced and thickened, then stir In half of the coriander and season to taste.
2. Heat the remaining oil in another frying pan and set over a medium to high heat. When the pan is hot, add the tofu and stir-fry for 4–5 minutes until golden and crispy all over. Remove and drain on kitchen paper.
3. Meanwhile, cook the rice according to the instructions on the packet.
4. Warm the taco shells and fill with the chickpea mixture and tofu. Sprinkle with the remaining coriander and top with some tomato salsa and yoghurt. Serve with lime wedges for squeezing plus the rice.

Or try this...
• Use canned black beans or red kidney beans instead of chickpeas.
• Add diced red or yellow peppers to the filling.
• Use smoky chipotle spice instead of chilli powder.
• Add crisp lettuce, tomatoes and diced red onion to the tacos.
• Substitute quinoa for the brown rice.

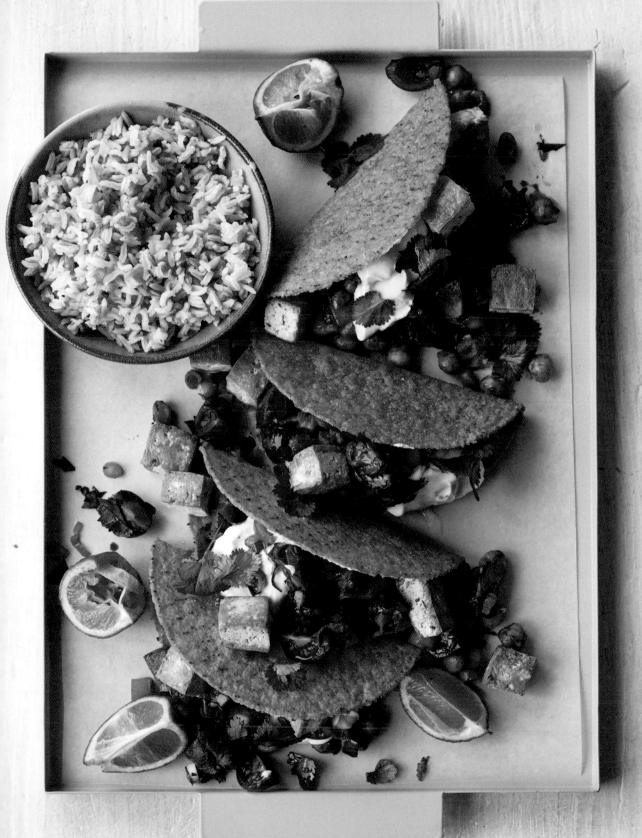

NACHOS WITH CHILLI BEEF

Serves 2
Prep: 15 minutes
Cook: 35–40 minutes

100g (3½oz) lower-calorie (or low-fat) tortilla chips
50g (2oz/½ cup) grated Cheddar cheese
1 red chilli, thinly sliced
6 black olives, stoned and sliced
a handful of coriander, chopped
4 tbsp 0% fat Greek yoghurt

Beef chilli:
spray olive oil
1 small onion, diced
2 garlic cloves, crushed
1 tsp chilli powder
1 tsp ground cumin
1 tsp ground cinnamon
1 tsp ground coriander
200g (7oz) extra-lean minced beef (5% fat max)
1 tbsp tomato paste
1 x 400g (14oz) can chopped tomatoes
1 x 200g (7oz) can red kidney beans, rinsed and drained
240ml (8fl oz/1 cup) hot beef stock
salt and black pepper

PER SERVING:
670 KCALS
39g PROTEIN
29g FAT
53.8g CARBS

Everyone loves nachos but my version, with lower-calorie cool tortilla chips and a really tasty low-fat chilli, is lighter than the usual. For a vegetarian option, make the chilli with canned jackfruit instead of beef. You could use shredded vegan cheese and dairy-free coconut yoghurt.

1. Make the beef chilli: lightly spray a saucepan with oil and set over a low to medium heat. Add the onion and garlic and cook for 8–10 minutes, stirring occasionally, until softened. Stir in the chilli powder and spices and cook for 1 minute.
2. Add the minced beef and cook for 4–5 minutes, stirring occasionally, until browned all over. Stir in the tomato paste, tomatoes, beans and stock. Bring to the boil, then reduce the heat and simmer for 15–20 minutes until the sauce reduces and thickens. Season to taste with salt and pepper.
3. Heat an overhead grill on high. Spread out the tortilla chips (with gaps in between) on a large baking tray. Sprinkle with three-quarters of the grated cheese and spoon the spicy beef chilli haphazardly over the top to expose some of the tortilla chips. Sprinkle with the chilli, olives and remaining cheese.
4. Cook under the hot grill for 5 minutes, or until the cheese melts and is golden brown. Divide between 2 serving plates and serve topped with the coriander and yoghurt.

Or try this...
- Serve with some guacamole, *pico de gallo* or hot salsa.
- Use black beans instead of red and jalapeno chillies.
- Add some diced avocado and sliced bottled red and yellow peppers.
- Drizzle with a hot sauce such as sriracha.

STIR-FRIED TERIYAKI SALMON

Serves 2
Prep: 15 minutes
Marinate: 10–15 minutes
Cook: 8 minutes

50ml (2fl oz/¼ cup) mirin
2 tbsp teriyaki sauce
200g (9oz) skinned salmon
   fillets, cut into strips
150g (5oz) flat rice noodles (dry
   weight)
2 tsp sesame oil
2.5cm (1in) piece fresh root
   ginger, peeled and grated
1 red or yellow pepper, deseeded
   and cut into strips
2 carrots, cut into thin
   matchsticks
4 spring onions, sliced diagonally
200g (7oz) pak choi, coarsely
   chopped
50g (2oz/½ cup) bean sprouts
grated zest and juice of 1 lime
1 tbsp black or white sesame
   seeds
a few sprigs of coriander,
   chopped

PER SERVING:

634 KCALS

31g PROTEIN

20.4g FAT

77g CARBS

This must be one of the healthiest and tastiest stir-fries ever. Salmon is packed with protein and heart-healthy omega-3 fats as well as vitamins A, B, D and E. Always buy wild salmon fillets in preference to farmed. They cost a little more but tend to have less saturated fat, fewer calories and more protein and essential minerals.

1. Stir together the mirin and teriyaki sauce in a shallow bowl. Add the salmon strips and coat in the marinade. Set aside for 10–15 minutes.
2. Cook the noodles according to the instructions on the packet.
3. Heat the sesame oil in a wok or deep frying pan over a medium to high heat. Add the salmon, reserving the marinade, and stir-fry gently for 3 minutes, or until browned all over.
4. Add the ginger, pepper, carrots, spring onions, pak choi and bean sprouts and stir-fry for 2–3 minutes, until just tender but slightly crunchy. Stir in the cooked egg noodles, lime juice and zest, reserved marinade and sesame seeds, and stir-fry for 1 minute.
5. Divide between 2 shallow serving bowls and serve immediately, sprinkled with coriander.

Tip: If you don't have any teriyaki sauce, use soy instead.

Or try this...
• Add a shredded chilli or some sweet chilli sauce.
• Add shredded kale, broccoli florets or mangetout.
• Try chicken, turkey or tofu instead of salmon.
• Use egg noodles instead of rice noodles.

BLACK COD WITH CRUNCHY SUGAR SNAPS

Serves 2
Prep: 15 minutes
Marinate: overnight
Cook: 15 minutes

2 x 200g (7oz) skinned thick
    cod fillets
125g (4½oz/generous ½ cup)
    wholegrain brown rice
spray oil
150g (5oz) sugar snap peas
2 tbsp teriyaki sauce
1 tsp white sesame seeds
2 tsp pickled ginger
2 spring onions, shredded

Marinade:
2 tbsp sake (Japanese rice wine)
2 tbsp mirin
4 tsp runny honey
2 tbsp white miso paste

PER SERVING:
550 KCALS
44g PROTEIN
8g FAT
64g CARBS

If you're like me and love Japanese food, you're going to be knocked out by this. You need to prepare the cod the day before you plan to eat it, so it absorbs the distinctive flavours of the miso marinade before cooking. It's so easy to make.

1. Make the marinade: put the sake, mirin and honey in a small saucepan over a high heat. Stir gently and when it comes to the boil, reduce the heat to low and add the miso. Stir until it dissolves then remove the pan from the heat.

2. When the marinade is cool, transfer it to a container large enough to accommodate the fish and add the cod fillets, turning them in the miso mixture until they are covered all over. Cover with a lid or cling film and marinate in the fridge overnight.

3. The following day, cook the brown rice according to the instructions on the packet.

4. When you're ready to cook the fish, pat it dry with kitchen paper. Lightly spray a large frying pan with oil and set over a medium to high heat. When the pan is hot, add the cod fillets and cook for 2–3 minutes, or until they brown underneath. Turn them over carefully and cook for 2–3 minutes on the other side.

5. Place the pan under a preheated hot overhead grill or in a preheated oven at 200°C (180°C fan/400°F/gas 6), and cook for 5–10 minutes, or until the cod is flaky and cooked right through.

6. Meanwhile, boil, steam or microwave the sugar snaps until just tender. Toss in the teriyaki sauce and sprinkle with sesame seeds.

7. Serve the black cod, garnished with the pickled ginger and spring onions, with the brown rice and sugar snaps.

Or try this...
• Serve with rice noodles drizzled with sesame oil.

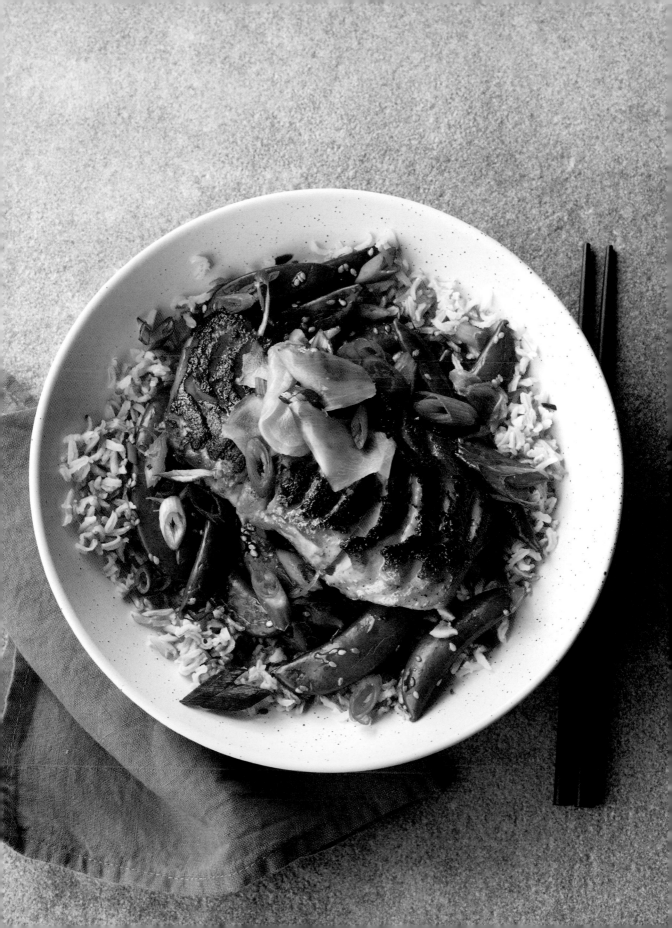

SNACKS

PEANUT BUTTER ENERGY BITES

Makes 24 bites
Prep: 15 minutes
Chill: at least 1 hour

50g (2oz/½ cup) dried apricots
75g (3oz/¾ cup) porridge oats
75g (3oz/⅓ cup) no-added-
   sugar crunchy or smooth
   peanut butter
2 tbsp sunflower seeds
1 tbsp runny honey
a few drops of vanilla extract
water or lemon juice, to mix
50g (2oz/generous ½ cup)
   dessicated coconut

PER BITE:
50 KCALS
1.5g PROTEIN
3.4g FAT
4.2g CARBS

These high-energy bites are delicious and really easy to make. And they're so nutritious – packed with protein, healthy carbs, vitamins and minerals. Because they're low GI, they're a great snack, releasing energy slowly and making you feel full – much healthier than a quick fix like a chocolate bar. Two bites are a 100 kcals snack.

1. Blitz the apricots, porridge oats, peanut butter, sunflower seeds, honey and vanilla in a blender or food processor until you have a rough, sticky paste. Add a little water or lemon juice, or even some more honey, to bind the mixture if it's too dry.
2. Divide into 24 small pieces and, using your hands, shape each one into a small ball. Roll the balls gently in the coconut until lightly coated all over.
3. Chill in the fridge for at least 1 hour to firm them up before transferring to an airtight container. They will keep well in the fridge for up to 10 days.

Tip: Make double the quantity and freeze one batch.

Note: Vegans can substitute maple or agave syrup for the honey.

Or try this...
- Use linseeds, flax seeds or chia seeds instead of sunflower seeds.
- Try another nut butter, e.g. cashew or almond.
- Add some cocoa or cacao powder for a chocolatey flavour.
- Add 2 tbsp vanilla- or chocolate-flavoured protein powder.
- Substitute Medjool dates for the apricots.

ENERGY PROTEIN BARS

Makes: 8 bars
Prep: 15 minutes
Cook: 15–20 minutes

100g (3½oz/1 cup) porridge oats
50g (2oz/½ cup) Medjool dates,
   stoned and chopped
50g (2oz/½ cup) dried ready-to-
   eat apricots, chopped
50g (2oz/½ cup) ready-to-eat
   prunes, chopped
2 tbsp chia seeds
1 ripe banana
2 tsp coconut oil
1 tsp runny honey
1 tsp ground cinnamon
a few drops of vanilla extract
cold water, to mix

PER BAR:
100 KCALS
3g PROTEIN
2.7g FAT
20g CARBS

I love these snack bars. They're a great pick-me-up at any time of day and a good source of energy and dietary fibre as well as protein. Take them to work or to college, or enjoy as an on-the-go snack when you're out exercising.

1. Preheat the oven to 180°C (160°C fan/350°F/gas 4). Line a shallow 20 x 20cm (8 x 8in) baking tin with baking parchment.
2. Put the porridge oats, dates, apricots, prunes and chia seeds in a bowl and mix well together. Mash the banana with a fork and add to the dried fruit and seeds.
3. Melt the coconut oil in a pan over a low heat and stir in the honey. Add to the oat and banana mixture with the cinnamon and vanilla and stir well. If the mixture is too dry and stiff, moisten it by adding enough cold water to make it soft and slightly sticky; if it's not firm enough, add more oats.
4. Transfer to the prepared tin and level the top, pressing it down with the back of a metal spoon. Bake in the preheated oven for 15–20 minutes, or until crisp and golden brown.
5. Remove from the oven and set aside to cool. While it's still warm, cut it into 8 bars. When they're completely cold, remove from the tin and store in an airtight container. The bars will stay fresh for up to 3–4 days.

Or try this...
• Vary the seeds: try pumpkin, linseeds, sesame or poppy seeds.
• Use different dried fruit, e.g. raisins or dried cranberries.
• Add some nut butter or dark chocolate chips.

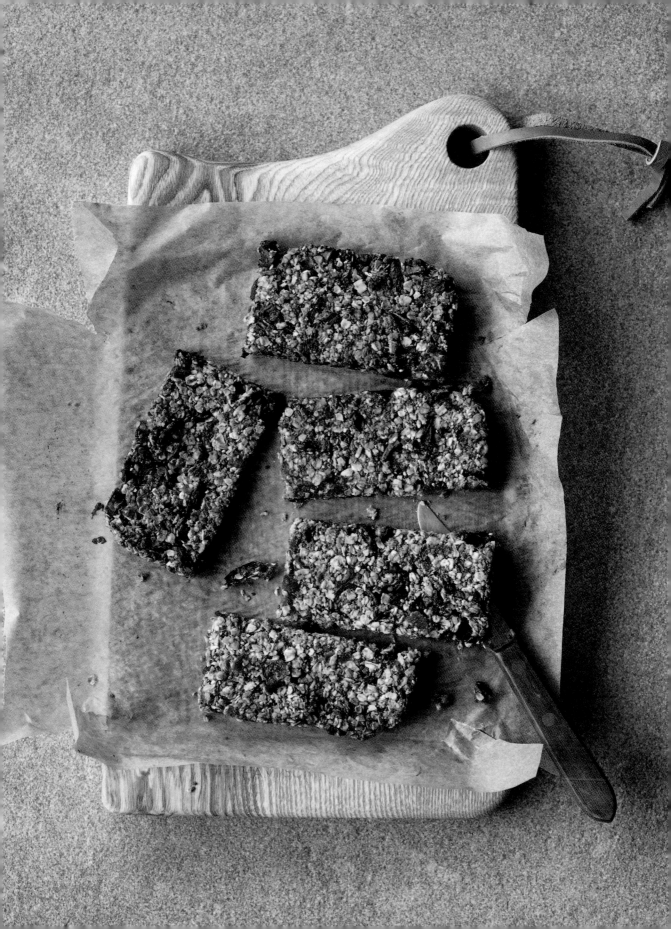

CHIA SEED CHOCOLATE POWER POTS

Serves 4
Prep: 10 minutes
Chill: overnight

1 banana, mashed
2 tsp nut butter, e.g. smooth
   peanut, almond or cashew
50g (2oz/4 tbsp) chocolate
   protein powder
300ml (½ pint/1¼ cups)
   unsweetened almond milk
6 tbsp chia seeds
100g (3½oz/1 cup) raspberries or
   blueberries
honey, for drizzling (optional)

PER POT:
155 KCALS
10.5g PROTEIN
8g FAT
9g CARBS

Chia seeds are a real powerhouse of nutrients, and when they are added to a liquid they swell up and thicken it – they can absorb up to 10 times their dry weight! I like to eat these little pots as a snack, but you can make them in 2 larger jars and have them for breakfast.

1. Put the mashed banana, nut butter, protein powder and milk in a blender and blitz until smooth.
2. Transfer to a bowl and stir in the chia seeds, distributing them evenly throughout the mixture – it should start thickening immediately. Pour into 4 small screw-top glass jars and cover with the lids or cling film. Leave to chill overnight in the fridge.
3. The mixture should be set by the following morning. Just before serving, top with the berries and drizzle with honey (if using).

Tip: You can use washed-out small glass yoghurt pots. If they don't have lids, cover with cling film.

Or try this...
• Top with chopped strawberries or peaches.
• Use skimmed milk, soya or coconut milk instead of almond milk.
• Sprinkle with coconut flakes.

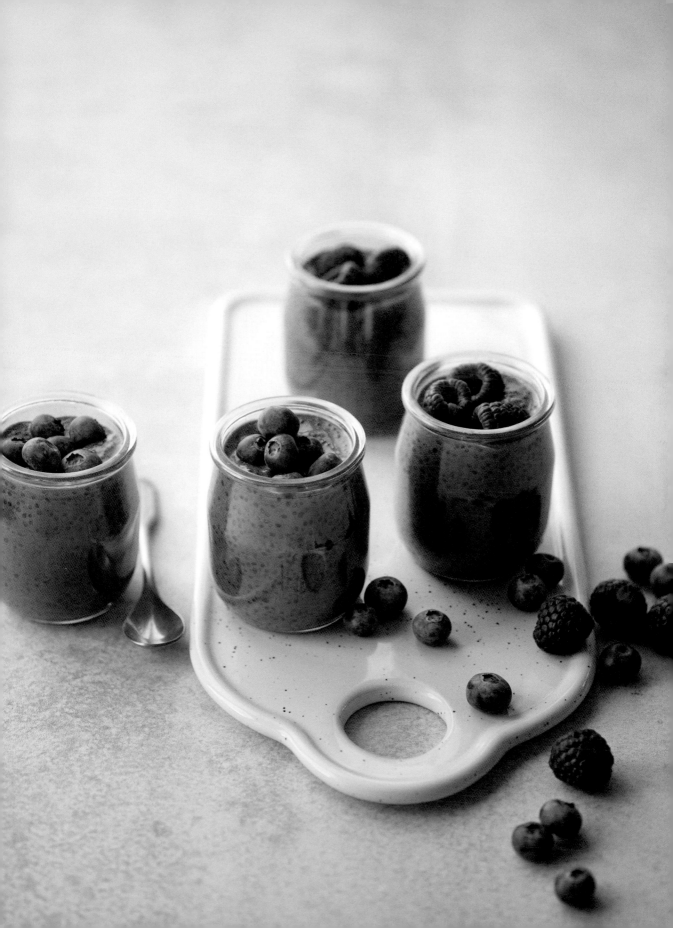

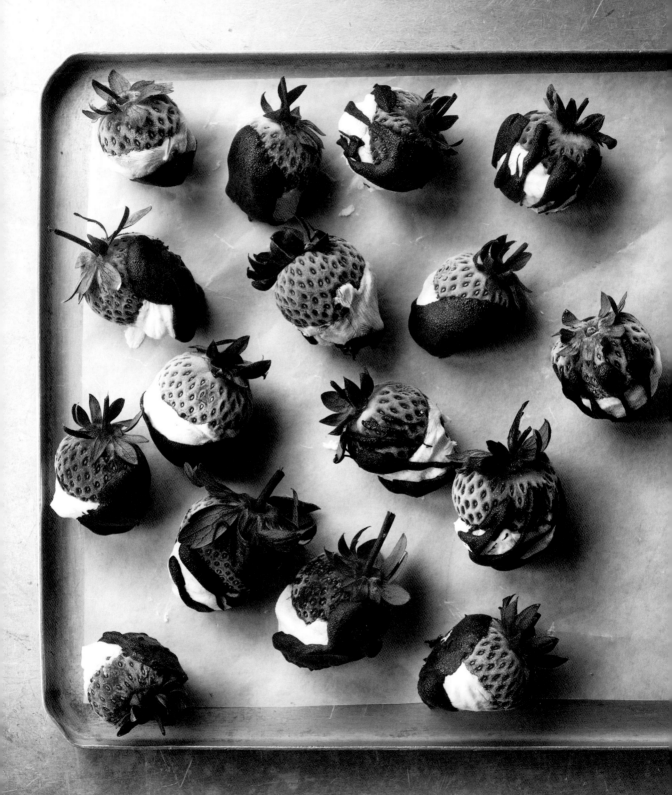

FROZEN YOGHURT-DIPPED STRAWBERRIES

Serves 4
Prep: 15 minutes
Freeze: 1¼–2¼ hours
Cook: 5 minutes

150g (5oz/generous ½ cup)
    0% fat Greek yoghurt
a few drops of vanilla extract
    (optional)
200g (7oz) strawberries (with
    stalks and leaves)
50g (2oz/scant ½ cup) dark
    chocolate chips

PER SERVING:

100 KCALS
5g PROTEIN
4g FAT
10g CARBS

Keep some of these yummy strawberries in the freezer for when you crave a sweet snack – they are much healthier than candy or a chocolate bar. And as a bonus, you can also serve them for a low-calorie dessert. Kids can't get enough of them!

1. Mix the yoghurt and vanilla extract (if using) in a bowl. Hold each strawberry by the stalk and leaves, lifting them up and away from the fruit, and dip them into the yoghurt. Leave a little area of red berry showing around the leaves at the top.
2. Place the strawberries, leaf-side down and tip-side up, on a wire rack that will fit into the freezer. Alternatively, place on a baking sheet lined with baking parchment.
3. Freeze for at least 1 hour or until the yoghurt is set and frozen. If you have any yoghurt left over, you can dip the frozen strawberries again to give them a second coating and return them to the freezer for 1 hour.
4. Put the chocolate chips in a heatproof bowl and suspend it over a pan of barely simmering water until the chocolate melts. Alternatively, melt the chocolate in a microwave.
5. Remove the frozen strawberries from the freezer and drizzle the melted chocolate over the top or dip the tips into it. Return the strawberries to the freezer for 15 minutes, or until set. Take them out of the freezer and leave in the fridge for 5–10 minutes before eating them.

Tip: These strawberries will keep well in the freezer for up to 1 month... if you can resist eating them in the first few days!

Or try this...
• Use blueberries instead of strawberries, coating them all over.
• Use milk chocolate chips instead of dark ones.

DIPPERS AND DIPS

You've always got low-calorie healthy snacks to hand if you keep at least a couple in the fridge. Here are some ideas to get you going. They're dead easy to make and taste awesome with some raw crunchy vegetable sticks – bin the crisps and tortilla chips and feast on celery, fennel, green, red and yellow peppers, broccoli and cauliflower florets, chicory and carrots instead.

LOW-FAT HUMMUS

Serves 6
Prep: 10 minutes

1 x 400g (14oz) can chickpeas
3 garlic cloves, crushed
1 tbsp tahini
juice of ½ lemon, plus extra
    to serve
½ tsp ground cumin
2 tbsp 0% fat Greek yoghurt
salt and freshly ground black
    pepper
paprika, for dusting

1. Drain the chickpeas, reserving 2–3 tablespoons of the liquid. Blitz the chickpeas, garlic, tahini, lemon juice and cumin in a blender to a thick, grainy purée.
2. Thin it with the reserved chickpea liquid, a little at a time, until it has the consistency of thick cream.
3. Transfer to a bowl or plastic container and stir in the yoghurt. Season to taste with salt and pepper, and dust lightly with paprika. Squeeze some lemon juice over the top (if you wish) and cover with a lid or cling film.

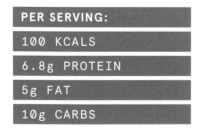

PER SERVING:

100 KCALS
6.8g PROTEIN
5g FAT
10g CARBS

SPEEDY SMOKED MACKEREL DIP

Serves 4
Prep: 5 minutes

2 x 80g (3oz) skinned smoked
    mackerel fillets
50g (2oz/¼ cup) light soft
    cheese
50g (2oz/¼ cup) 0% fat Greek
    yoghurt
1 tsp horseradish sauce
a good squeeze of lemon juice
a few sprigs of parsley, chopped
freshly ground black pepper

1. Put all the ingredients in a blender or food processor and blitz
   until smooth and creamy.
2. Transfer to a bowl or plastic container and cover with a lid or
   cling film. Keep in the fridge and serve as a dip or spread.

PER SERVING:

150 KCALS

11.7g PROTEIN

10g FAT

1.6g CARBS

SMASHED BEAN DIP

Serves 6
Prep: 10 minutes

2 x 400g (14oz) cans beans,
    e.g. cannellini, haricot,
    butterbeans, rinsed and
    drained
50g (2oz/¼ cup) light soft
    cheese
4 tbsp 0% fat Greek yoghurt
4 spring onions, diced
2 garlic cloves, crushed
grated zest and juice of 1 lemon
salt and fresh ground black
    pepper
sweet chilli sauce, for drizzling

1. Blitz one can of beans in a blender with the soft cheese, yoghurt,
   onions, garlic, lemon zest and juice. Transfer to a bowl or plastic
   container.
2. Coarsely mash the remaining beans with a fork or potato
   masher and stir into the bean dip. Season with salt and pepper,
   then drizzle with chilli sauce, or swirl it in.

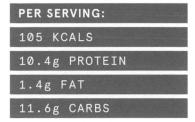

PER SERVING:

105 KCALS

10.4g PROTEIN

1.4g FAT

11.6g CARBS

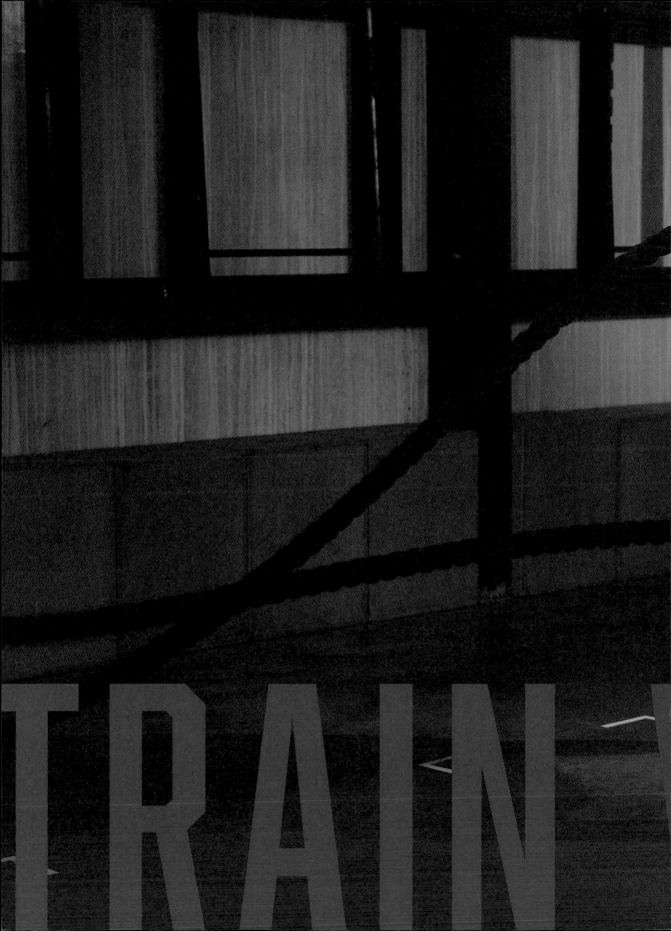

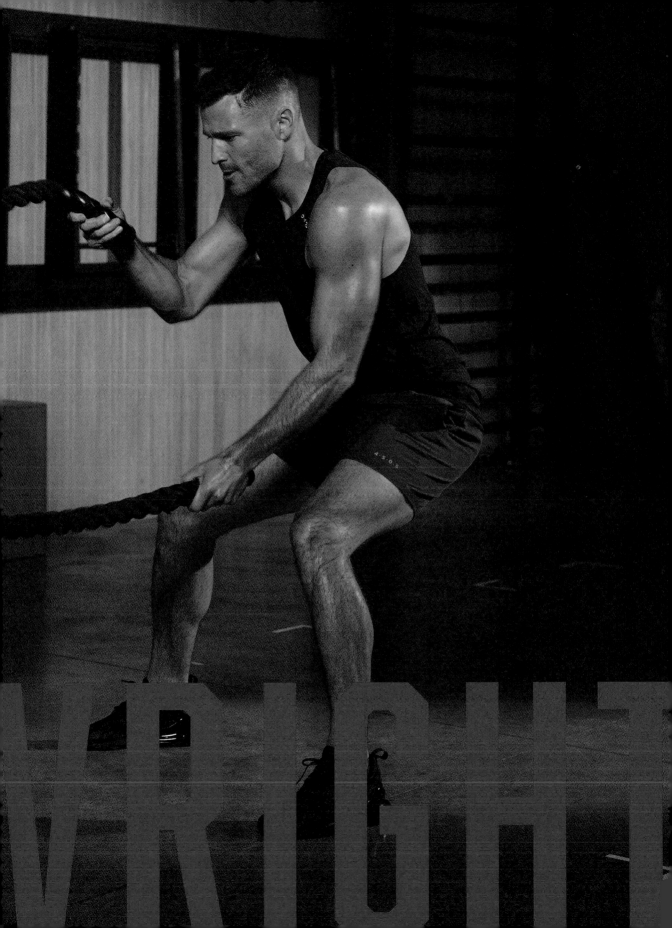

CHAPTER 5 – THE WORKOUTS

Alright, you've made it! This is my favourite part of the Get Fit, Get Healthy, Get Happy journey and soon enough it's going to be yours too. Exercise is such an important part of my life because I know the power regular exercise has on every aspect of what I do. That's why I get so excited when people come to me for advice at the start of a fitness journey and it is what inspired me to write this book. I am genuinely passionate about the difference exercise can make to your confidence, your health, your productivity, your relationships and your overall happiness. Honestly I'm not exaggerating when I say that the positive impacts of regular exercise are endless. If that's not enough to make you excited about starting this plan I don't know what is.

Over the next six weeks I am going to show you how to incorporate home workouts into your life through my favourite ways of training, a mixture of HIIT (High Intensity Interval Training), boxing, bodyweight strength and LISS (Low Intensity Steady State) exercise. I have designed these workouts so that every single one is completely different – you'll never do the same workout twice and you'll never get bored. Paired with the Eat Wright meals, this training plan has been specifically designed to help you smash your goals, whether that's to lose weight, build strength or improve your focus. Get prepared to start the Train Wright section of your journey to a fitter, healthier, happier you.

HOW IT WORKS

For the next six weeks I will lay out a training plan for you to follow. The idea of the six-week plan is that it will kickstart your journey in forming healthier habits as well as getting you fitter, stronger, healthier and well on your way to reaching your fitness goals.

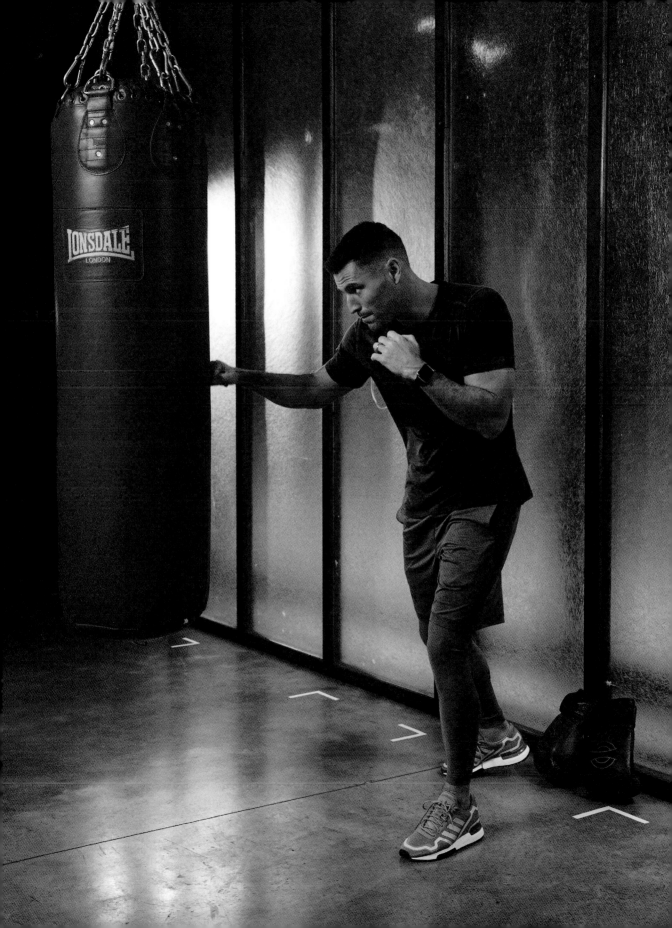

THE PLAN

Each week you will complete four high-intensity workouts, each one lasting between 25 and 30 minutes. You will complete one LISS training day and will have two rest days.

Alongside your exercise plan, you will be eating three delicious meals from the food chapter (see pages 52–119) and one snack every day, along with drinking at least two litres of water.

LOW INTENSITY STEADY STATE (LISS) DAYS

I'm a big fan of home workouts, because I know how effective they can be at getting you amazing results in a short space of time without having to leave your living room. But I also believe in just moving more. Some of the days I burn the most calories aren't the days I fit in a workout, but the days I'm really busy and on my feet all day. That's why I was so keen to include one LISS day a week in your training plan. LISS simple means 'Low Intensity Steady State' training. While a workout usually sees us push ourselves to the max, LISS is continuous movement but at a lower intensity. This can be fast-paced walking, cycling, swimming, a slow jog or even a yoga class or much lower-intensity workout. So, instead of pushing yourself to that high level of work for short bursts, on LISS days I want you to aim for a lower level of physical work but for a longer time of at least an hour in total. You can plan two half-hour walks, one hour-long walk, an hour slow cycle or an hour yoga class – whatever movement it is, do it with meaning but enjoy the lower-intensity style of activity.

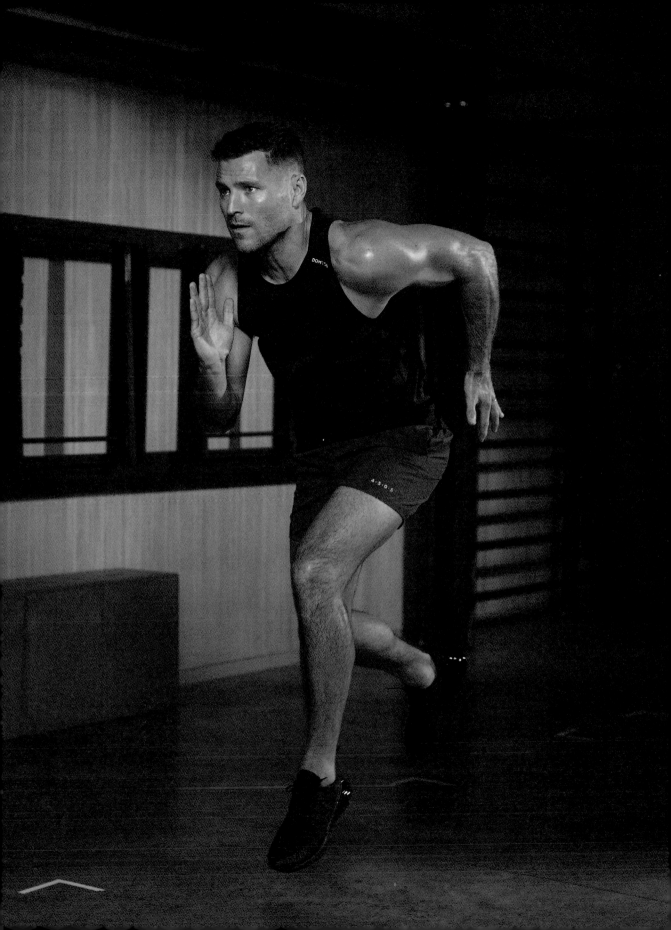

Always perform a warm-up before exercising. This part is so important if you are going to be working out at a high intensity. I've put together my favourite warm-up moves for you to complete before every workout, but if you have other moves you know work well for you, feel free to add those in at the end too. Warming up isn't just about preventing injury or muscle soreness, warming up also means we prepare our bodies for the workout, helping us to work harder and more effectively during the workout itself. If we don't switch our muscles on, we can't expect them to work to their max. These exercises always get my muscles fired up and my body warm and ready to work out. Perform each one for the time given.

MID-RANGE HIGH KNEES ON THE SPOT

Start in a standing position and take a gentle jog on the spot.

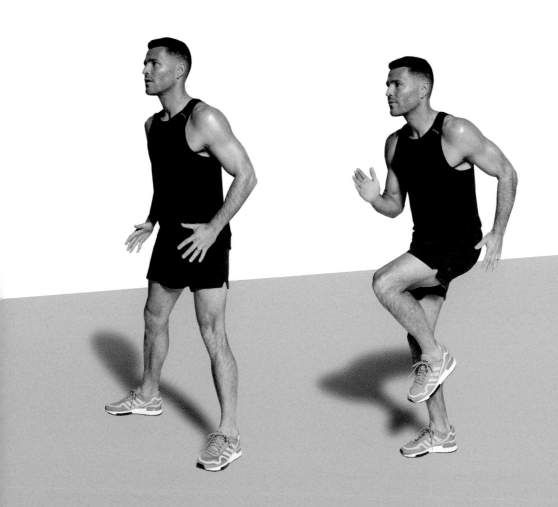

⏱ **30 SECONDS**

STANDING SQUAT

Squat down, sending your bum backwards and keeping your knees in line. Return to a standing position by pushing down through your heels.

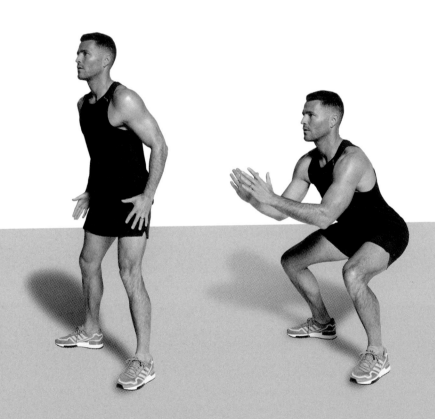

⏱ **20 SECONDS**

SLOW SKIER JUMP HOLD

Start in a standing position then power off the left foot and jump laterally (sideways) to the right and kick the left foot behind you. Hold and balance here for a second before swapping legs.

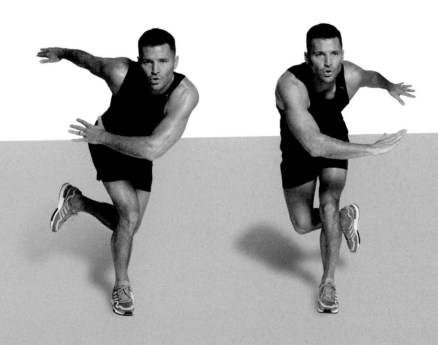

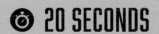 **20 SECONDS**

PLANK LUNGE REACH OPEN

Start in a high plank position, then step your left foot forward next to your left hand. Slowly lift your left arm up and reach it to the ceiling. Return it to the floor and step the left foot back to plank. Repeat on the right side.

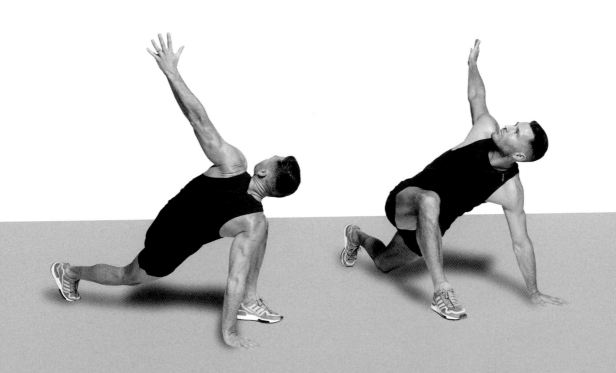

⏱ **30 SECONDS, SWAPPING BETWEEN EACH SIDE**

JAB-CROSS BOXING

Start in a boxer's stance (see page 188), then punch each arm forward one after the other.

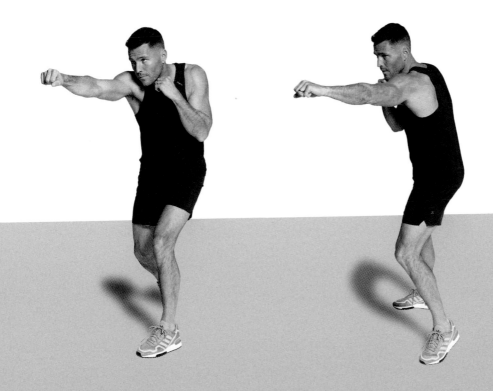

⏱ **20 SECONDS**

STANDING TWISTS

Start in a standing position, twist your upper body to the left and, as you do this, twist the right leg to allow the body to come fully round to the side. Repeat in the opposite direction.

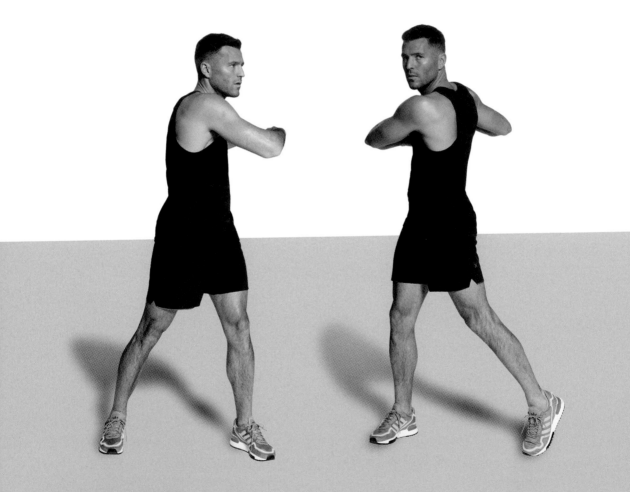

⏱ **20 SECONDS**

LEAN-FORWARD ELBOW-MOBILITY SWINGS

Start in a standing position, feet just wider than hip-width apart. Lean forward, then perform big circles of the shoulders, with the elbows bent.

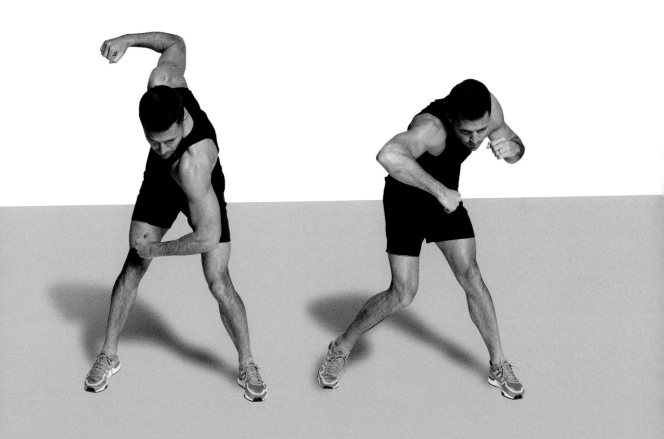

⏱ **20 SECONDS**

30-MINUT
HOME
WORKOUT

MOUNTAIN CLIMBERS

Start in a high plank position. Look down towards your hands and keep your back flat. From here, drive your left knee towards your chest then bounce to swap legs so your right knee comes towards the chest. Repeat as fast as possible.

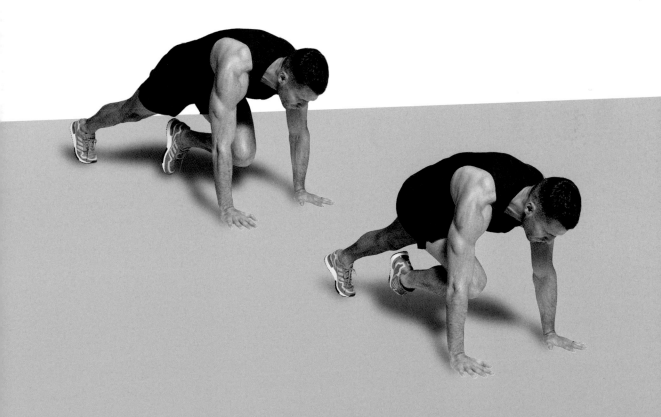

SQUATS

Start in a standing position with feet just wider than hips. From here, sit your bum back and bend your knees to take you into a squat position, with your arms bent and palms at the back of your head. Push back up to standing.

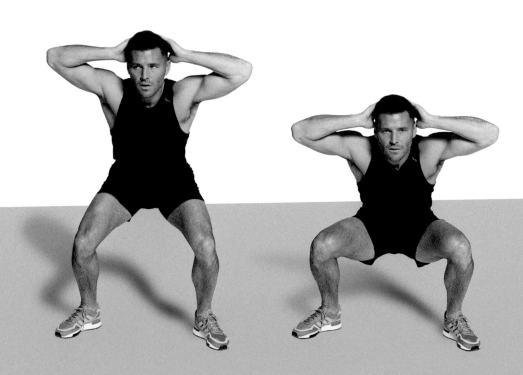

LOW PLANK HOLD

With arms bent and elbows under shoulders, rest your weight on your forearms and bring your body into a straight line, with your toes taking your weight. Hold.

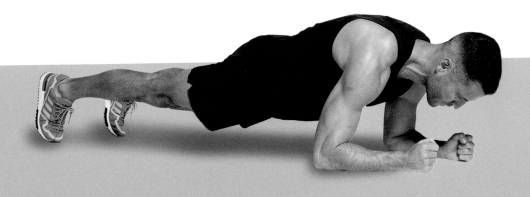

FULL STAR JUMPS

Start in a standing position, then jump both feet together and bend your knees to bring you into a narrow squat. Bring your hands down. From here, explode up and bring both feet quickly out wide and, at the same time, bring both hands up above your head. As you come back to land, bring your feet together and land back into the narrow squat. Repeat.

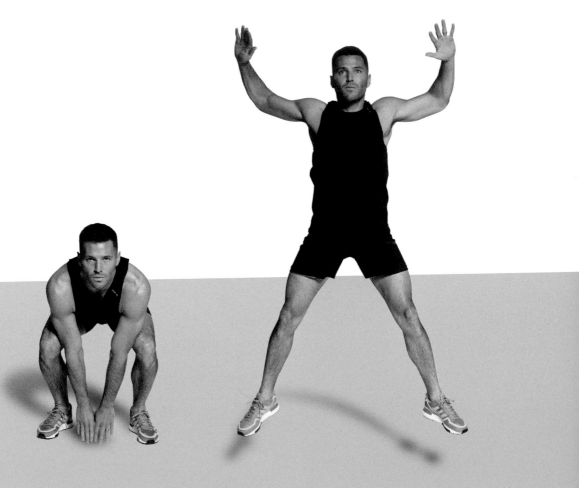

KNEE SLAMS

Stand on the spot, engage your core muscles and lift both hands above your head. Drive the left knee up with power and bring your arms down to your sides. Add in a little bounce as you repeat, this time lifting the right knee. The key here is to go as fast as you can.

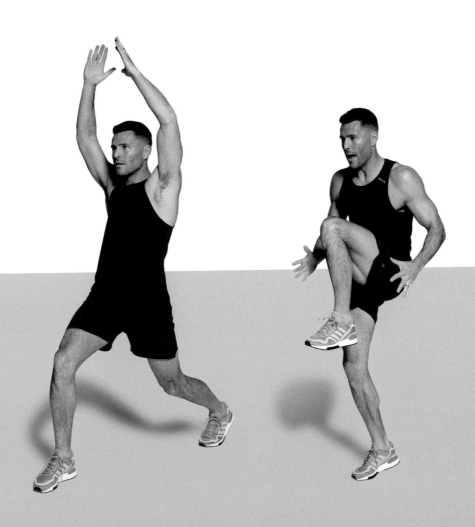

MOUNTAIN CLIMBERS TO PLANK JACKS

Start in a high plank position. Look down towards your hands and keep your back flat. From here, drive your opposite knee to your opposite elbow, once on each side, then jump both feet out wide and then back to centre, twice, before returning to the mountain climbers.

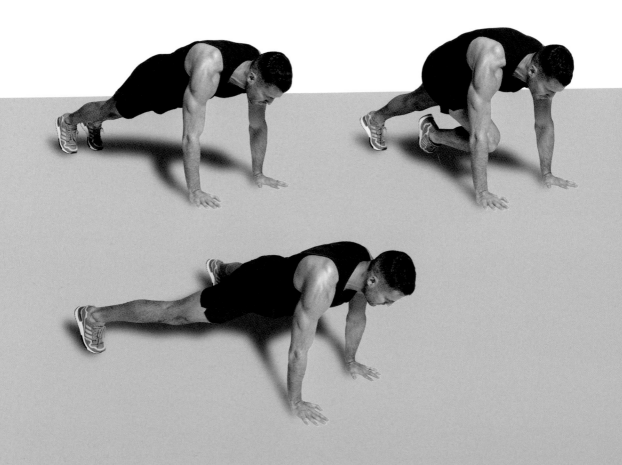

PRESS-UPS

Start in a high plank position with your hands on the floor, wrists positioned under your shoulders. While engaging your core muscles, slowly lower your chest towards the floor by bending your elbows, keeping your gaze between your hands, and making sure your lower back doesn't dip down. With power, push back up to the start position.

Note: If you are a beginner, drop down to your knees and bring the weight forward over your wrists. While engaging your core muscles, slowly lower your chest towards the floor by bending your elbows, keeping your gaze between your hands and making sure your lower back doesn't dip down. With power, push back up to the start position.

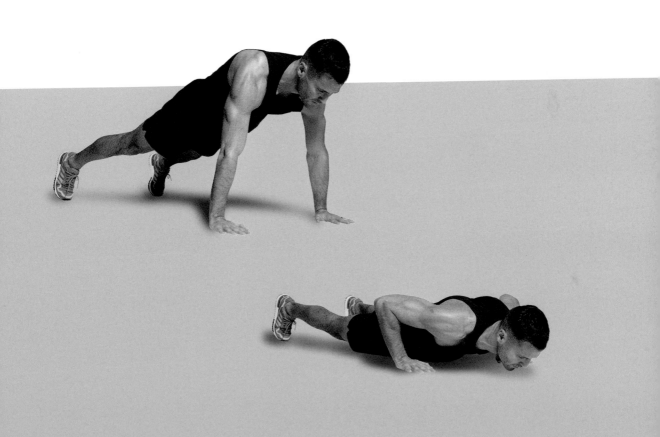

SPEED SKATERS

Start in a standing position, with both arms straight and chest up, then power off the left foot, jump laterally (sideways) to the right and kick the left foot behind you. Immediately power off the right foot and repeat the movement on the opposite side.

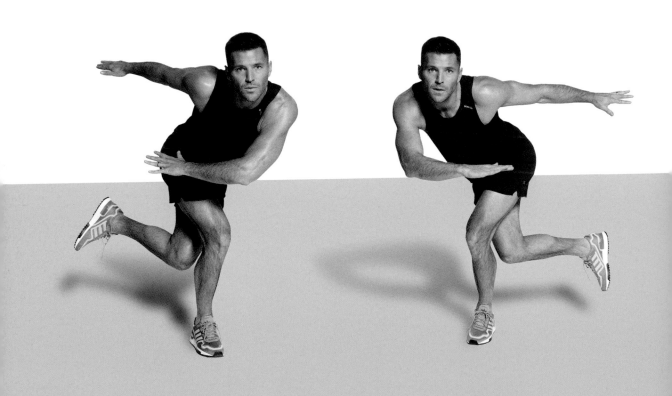

SPRINT ON THE SPOT

Start in a standing position, then drive one knee up in front of you as high as you can, to hip height. Quickly switch over so your opposite knee drives up, and continue these movements as fast as you can, as if sprinting on the spot.

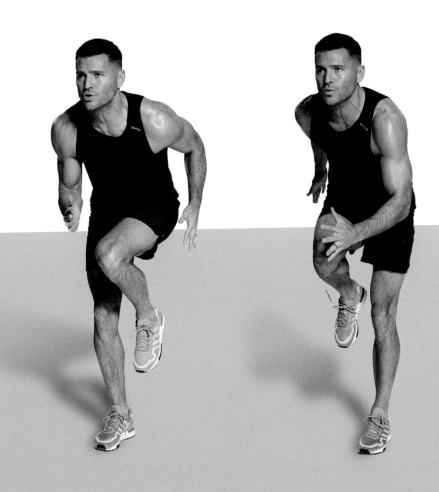

SQUAT JUMP KICKS

Start in a standing position with your feet just wider than shoulder-width apart.

Bend your knees and send your bum back and down into a squat position, keeping your chest lifted. Push off the floor and jump into the air. Land back in a squat position, taking care to prevent your knees from rolling inwards when you land.

From here, power up off your left foot to bring yourself to standing, then kick your left leg forward in front of you. Return the left foot to where it was before and repeat from the top. On each set, alternate which leg kicks forward.

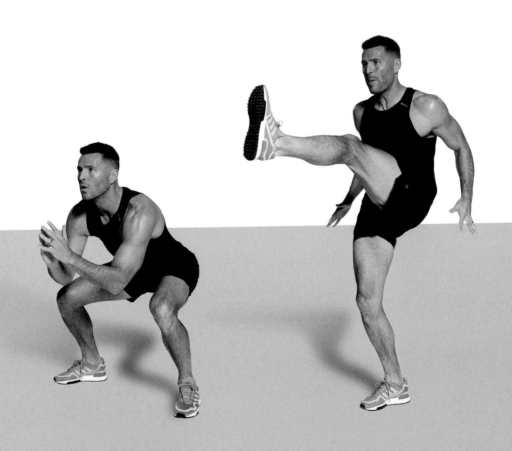

KNEE DRIVES

Start in a standing position with one leg stepped back behind the other. Lean forward over the front leg and bring your arms up in line with your head. From here, drive the knee of the back leg forward and at the same time bring both arms down, with power. Return quickly to the start position and repeat.

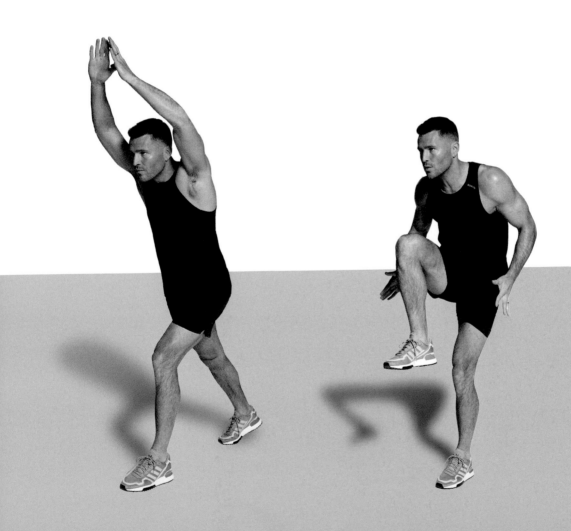

NSEW (NORTH SOUTH EAST WEST) SQUAT JUMPS

Start in a standing position, then jump forward and bend your knees to land in a squat position. From here, jump backwards to the start by powering through the legs and landing by bending the knees. Repeat this movement but this time to 'south' behind you, then the 'east' to the right of you, then the 'west' to your left, each time returning to the start position. Repeat.

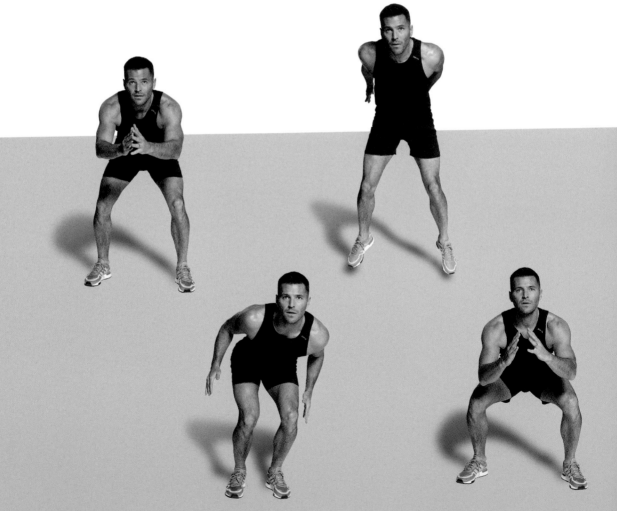

HOPS

Stand on one leg. Once you have your balance, hop forward then back while staying on one leg.

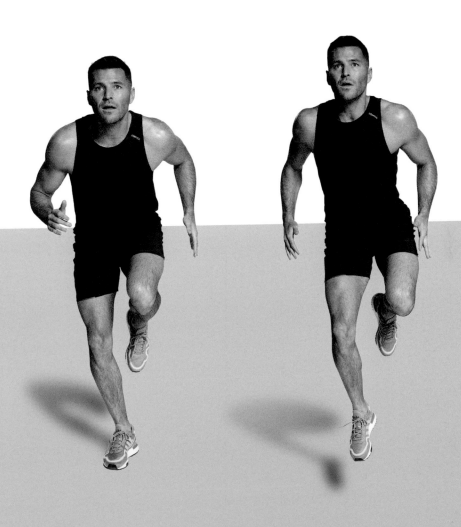

KNEES-UP PUNCH-OUTS

Start in a standing position, then drive one knee up, then the other, as high as you can. At the same time, punch your fists out in front of you one at a time, as fast as you are able, to punch and sprint on the spot at the same time.

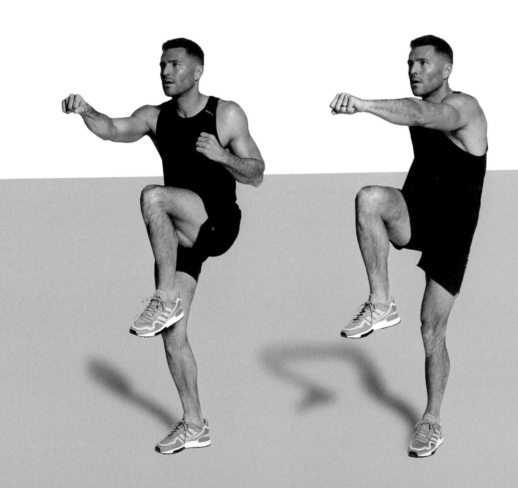

JUMP JACK STEP-OUTS

Start in a standing position, then jump both feet out wide and bring your hands above your head into a star jump. From here, return to the starting position then jump one foot forward and one back and bring opposite arm forward and the other arm back. Return to the start and repeat.

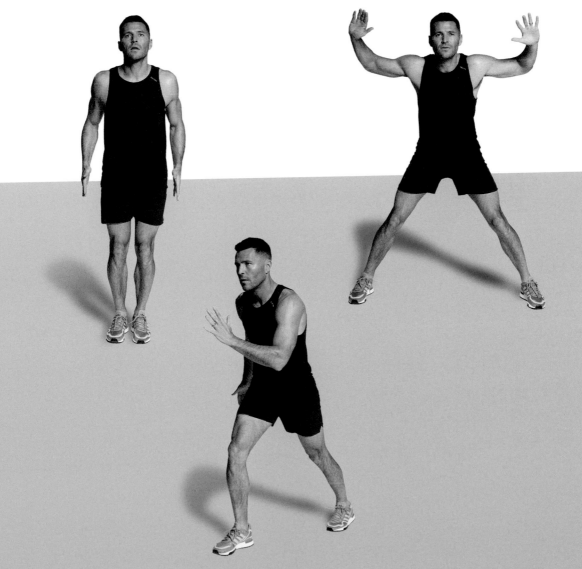

SQUAT KNEE TO ELBOW

Start in a standing position with feet wider than hips. Sit your bum back and bend your knees to take you into a squat position, and bend your arms to lightly place your fingers on either side of your head. Drive up to standing while at the same time lifting your left foot off the floor and driving the left knee up to meet the right elbow. Plant the left foot back to the floor and repeat on the opposite side.

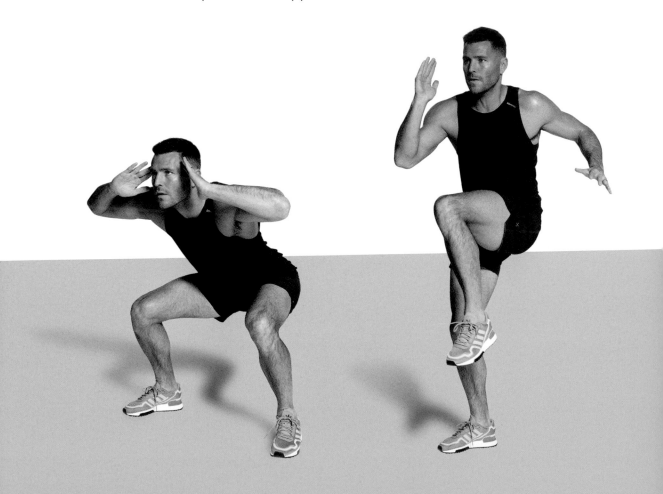

TOE TAPS

Start in a standing position, jump and bring the toe of your left foot to tap directly in front of you. Quickly swap the feet so the right toe is tapped in front of you. Repeat as fast as you can.

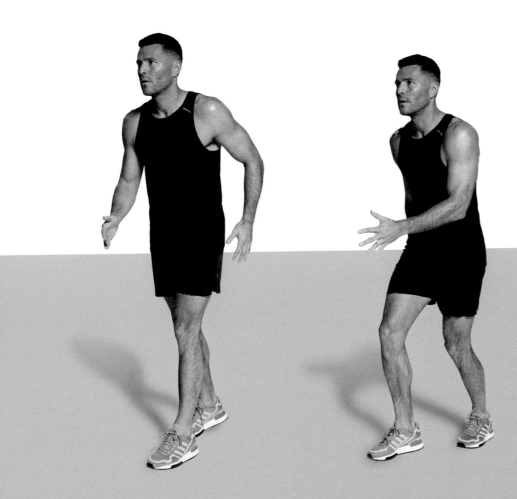

BROAD JUMP, JUMP BACK

Start in a standing position, jump forward and bend your knees to land in a squat position. From here, jump backwards to the start position by powering through the legs and land by bending the knees. Use your arms to create momentum by swiping them forward.

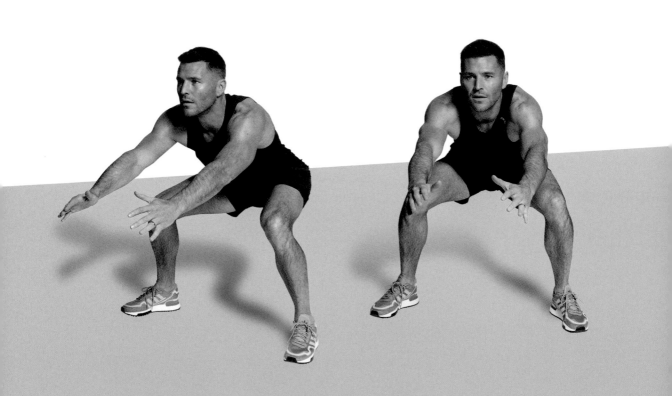

SHOOT-THROUGHS

Start on your hands and knees then push through your toes to lift your knees so they are hovering above the floor. Lift your right hand off the floor and, as you do this, twist your body to the right, reaching your arm to the ceiling, and lift your left leg to bring it underneath you to kick to the right-hand side. Return to the start then repeat on the opposite side.

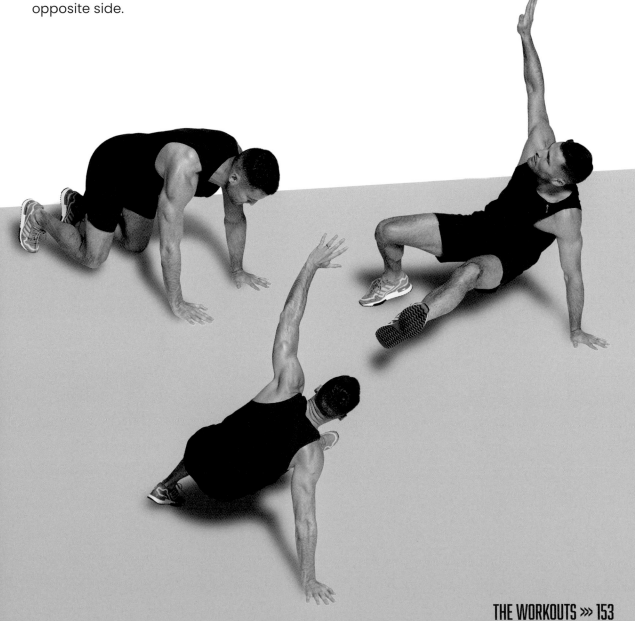

SPRAWLS

Start in a high plank position with your hands placed under shoulders and your body in a straight line. From here, jump the feet wide next to your hands and then lift your hands and bring your head and chest up as you sit your weight back into your heels. Plant your hands back down and jump back to the plank position. Repeat.

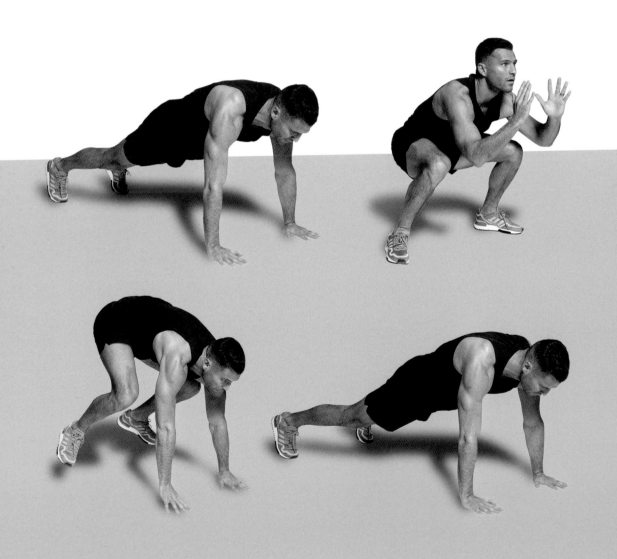

HALF BURPEES

Start in a standing position, then bring both your hands to the floor. Jump both feet back into a plank then jump both feet back to the top and stand up and jump. Repeat.

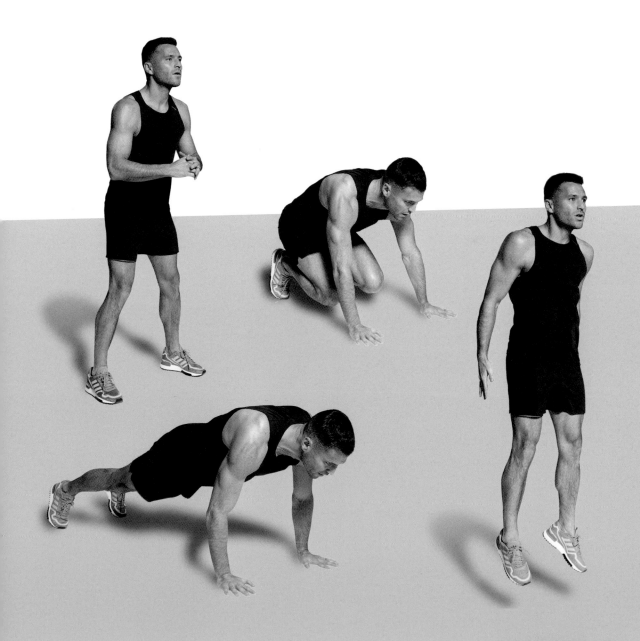

SINGLE-ARM BURPEES

Start in a standing position, tuck your left arm back and bring your right hand to the floor. Jump both feet back into a single-arm plank then jump both feet back to the top, stand up and jump. Repeat with the opposite arm.

Note: This exercise is for advanced exercisers. If you are a beginner or intermediate, substitute this for a regular burpee (see page 185).

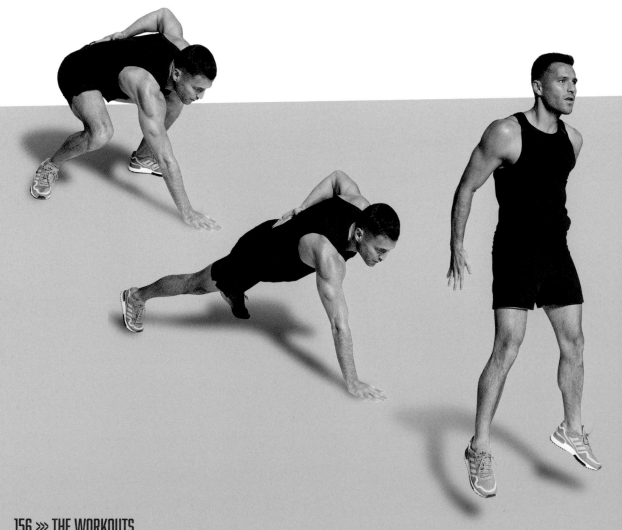

INCHWORMS

Start in a standing position, then roll your body down to bring your hands to the floor in front of you, bending your knees. From here, walk your hands forward to bring yourself into a high plank position. Hold for a second before walking both hands back towards the feet and rolling your body back up to a standing position. Repeat.

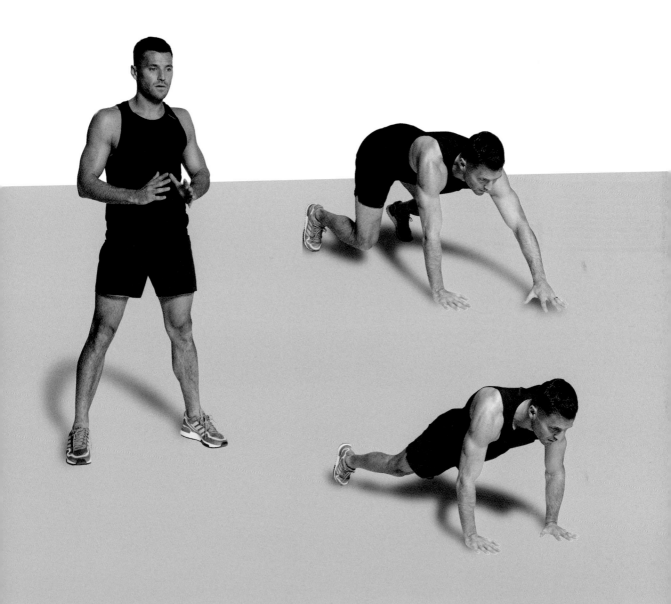

REVERSE PLANK KNEE-INS

Sit on the floor with both legs straight out in front of you. Plant your hands on the floor next to your hips and push down into your heels to bring your bum off the floor. From here, lift your right leg up and drive your right knee towards your chest. Return it back to the floor and repeat with the left leg.

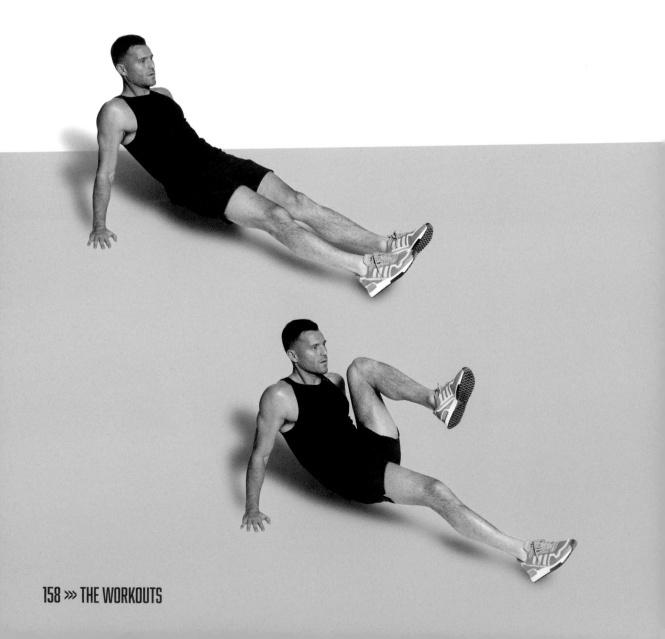

DOUBLE CROSSOVER SQUATS

Start in a standing position, then sit your bum back and bend your knees to come into a squat position. From here, jump up and cross your legs over in mid-air and land in a cross position. From here, jump the feet out to a wide stance, then jump and cross them over again, this time the opposite way round. For the last time, jump up and this time land back in the squat position. Repeat.

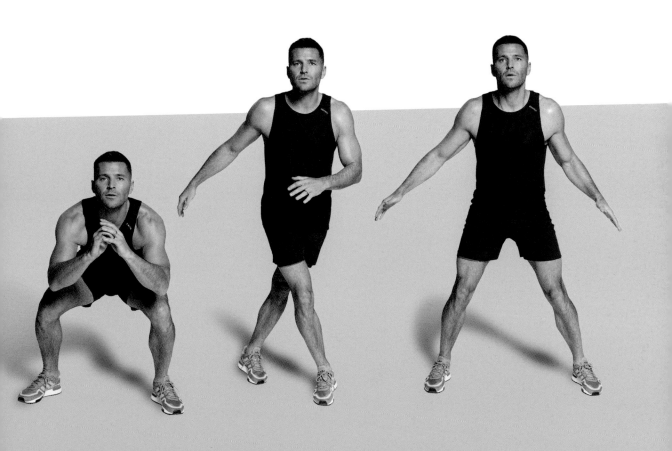

LOW-WALK TWISTS

Sit your bum back and bend your knees to bring you into a squat position. Staying low, step the left leg forward directly in line with the right then immediately step the right leg forward in line with the left. Walk forward in a low squat while twisting the body. Once you reach the end of the room, turn round and repeat on the way back.

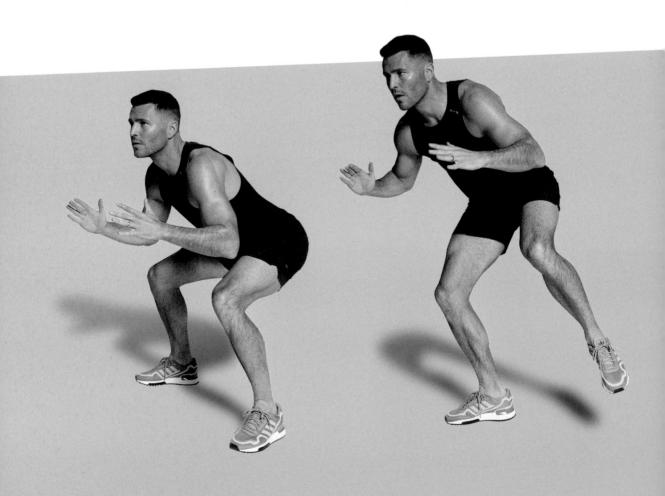

PRESS UP, REACH OUT

Perform a press-up (see page 141) then, as you reach the top position, lift one arm while balancing on the other and reach it directly forward at head height. Return it to the plank position then perform another press-up and this time lift the other arm.
NOTE: If you are a beginner, drop down to your knees.

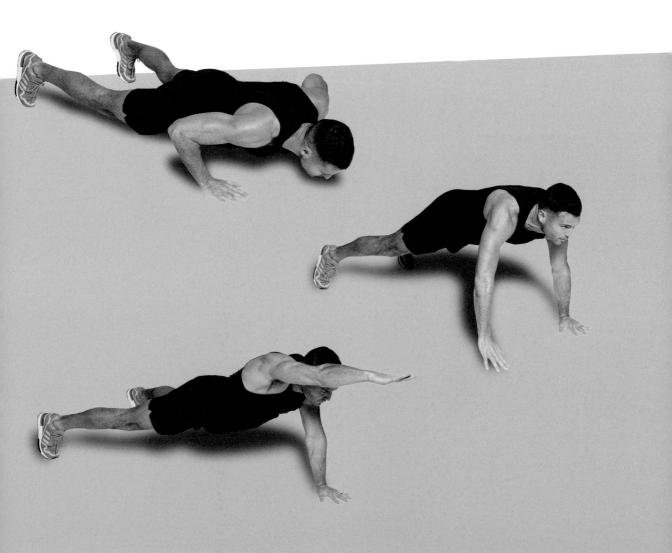

FROG SQUATS

Start in a standing position, then step your right leg out to the side while bending your left leg. At the same time bring your right hand down to touch the left ankle and shoot your left arm out to the side. Quickly jump and swap your legs over to repeat on the other side.

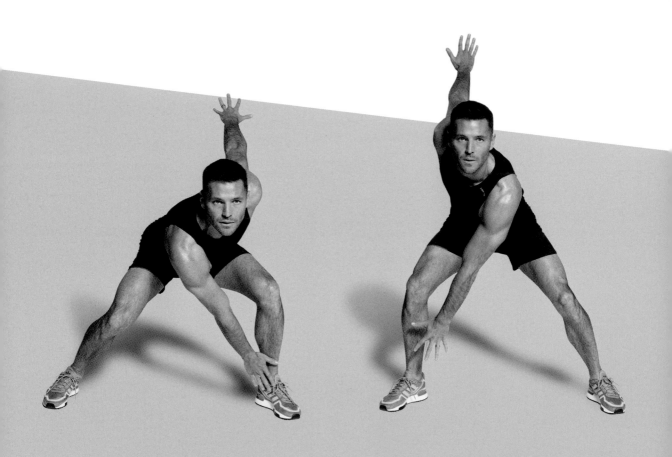

RUNNING-MAN LUNGE JUMPS

Start in a standing position, then jump one foot forward and one back and bring opposite arms forward and back. Jump up and swap the feet round. Once you have completed the two shuffles, jump up and this time land in a low lunge position by bending the knee of the back leg down and bending the front knee so your foot is flat on the floor. Jump up and swap the legs over in mid-air to land in a lunge on the opposite side.

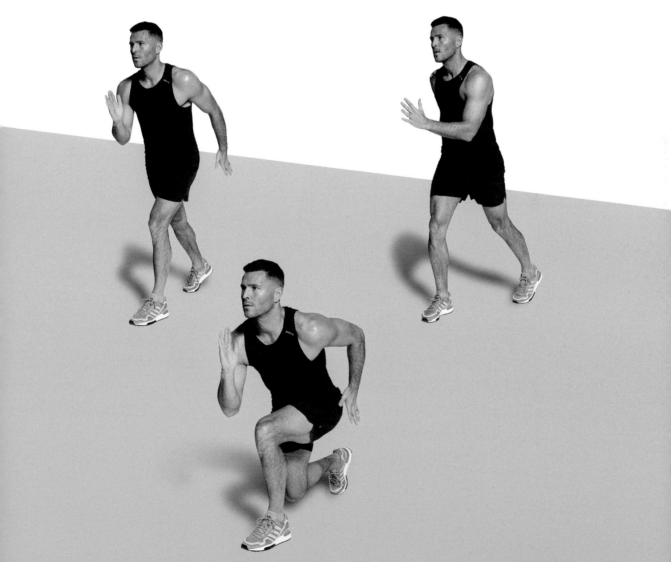

KNEE-SLAM BURPEES

Start in a standing position and bring both hands to the floor. Jump both feet back into a plank then jump both feet back to the top and stand up. As you stand, bring your left knee up to a standing knee slam. Quickly return to standing position and repeat from the top, this time crunching in the right knee.

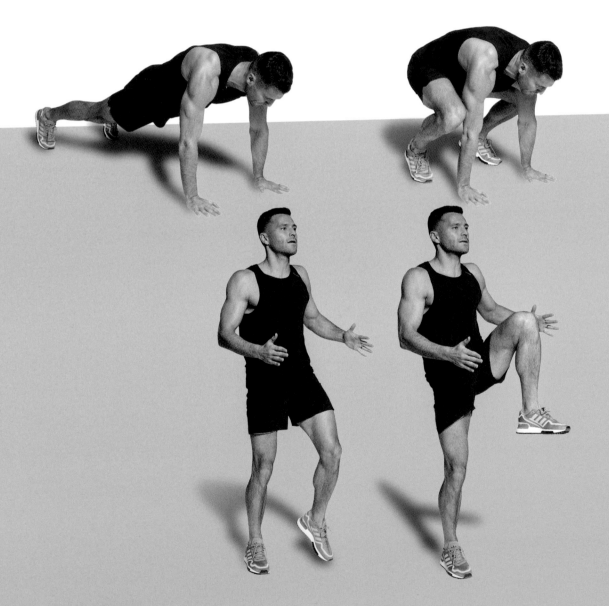

SINGLE-LEG DONKEY KICKS

Start on all fours then push into your toes to lift the knees. From this position, kick the heel of your right foot to your bum, then quickly swap over so the left foot kicks your bum. Repeat.

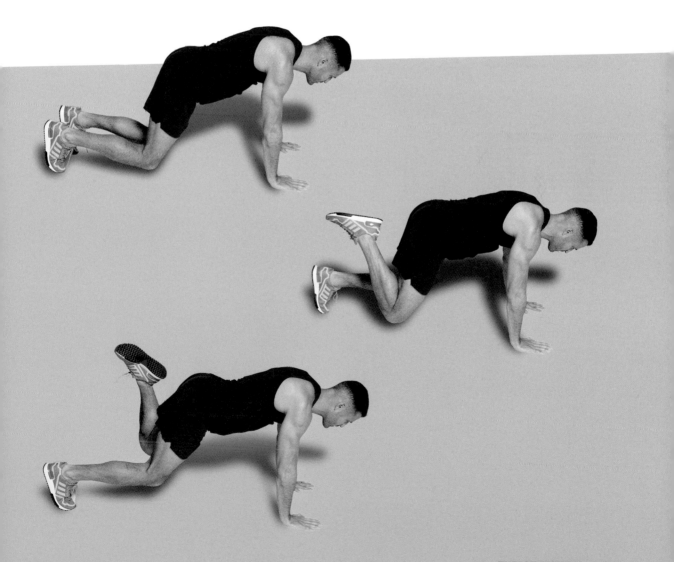

DONKEY KICKS

Start on all fours then push into your toes to lift the knees. From this position, let your weight come forward and kick both heels of your feet to your bum, before landing back in the start position. Repeat.

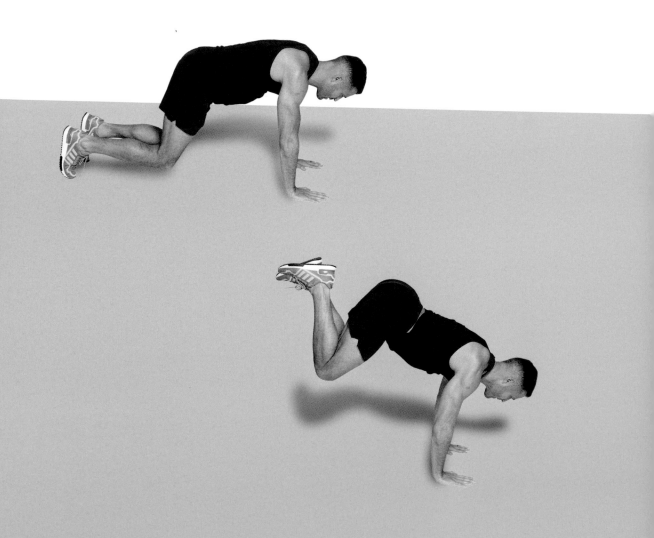

SQUAT POP TWISTS

Start in a standing position with feet just wider than hips. From here, sit your bum back and bend your knees to take you into a squat position. Push into your heels to jump up and, as you do, twist the body to the right so you land in a twist position. Jump back to the centre and land back down in a squat then repeat, this time twisting to the left.

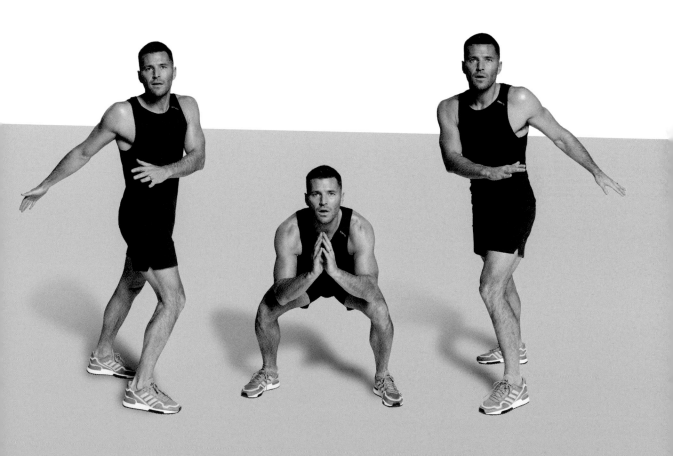

CROSS-BODY MOUNTAIN CLIMBERS

From a high plank position look down towards your hands and keep your back flat, then drive opposite knee to opposite elbow, alternating knee and elbow, as fast as possible.

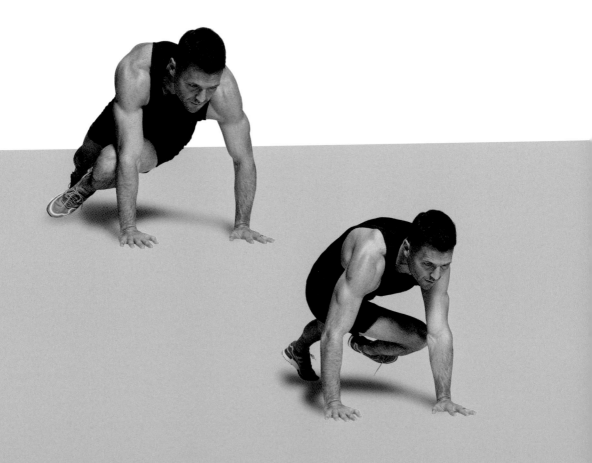

180-DEGREE SQUAT JUMPS

Start in a standing position with feet just wider than hips. From here, sit your bum back and bend your knees to take you into a squat position. Push down into your heels to jump up and, as you jump, twist your body to turn 180 degrees in mid-air and land in a squat facing the opposite direction. Repeat.

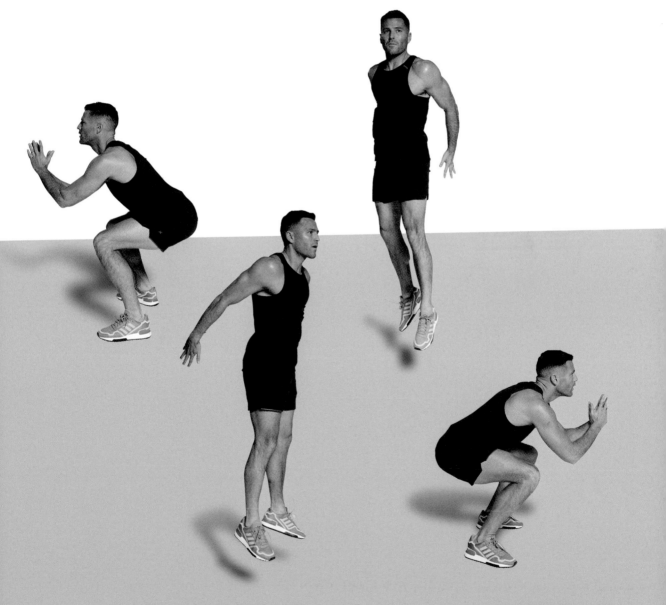

FORWARD BEAR CRAWL

Start on all fours then push into your toes to lift the knees. From this position, lift your left hand and reach it forward while, at the same time, lifting your right foot and stepping it forward. Stay low in a crawl position throughout this movement, then repeat on the opposite side, moving forward.

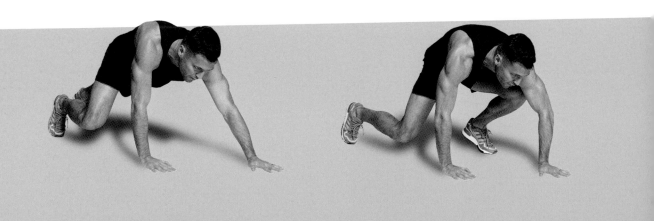

SQUAT TO 4 HIGH KNEES

Start in a standing position with feet just wider than hips. From here, sit your bum back and bend your knees to take you into a squat position. Push down into your heels to bring you up to standing, then perform four quick high knees, first driving the right knee up, then jumping and swapping mid-air to bring the left knee up. Repeat.

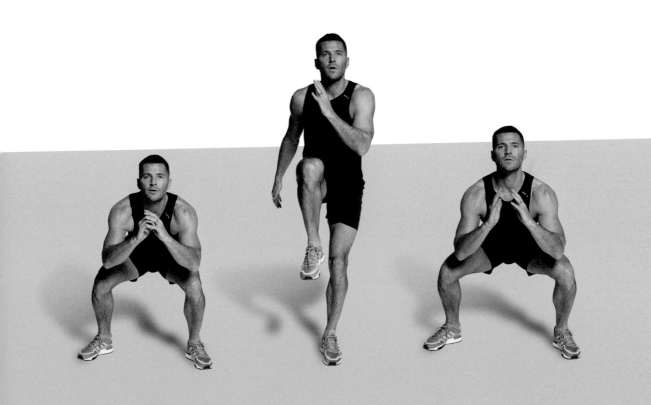

LUNGE PULSES

Start in a standing position then step your right foot back behind you. Bend both knees to bring you down into a lunge. From here, semi-straighten both legs and push through the feet to bring you into a high lunge before bending both knees to bring you down again. Repeat.

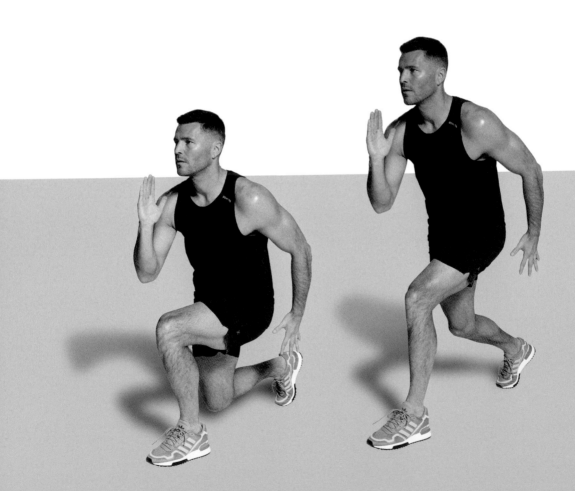

HALF-BURPEE SQUAT PULSES

Start in a standing position, then bring both hands to the floor. Jump both feet back into a high plank then jump both feet back to the top and stand up. Immediately sit your bum back into a squat. Stand and repeat.

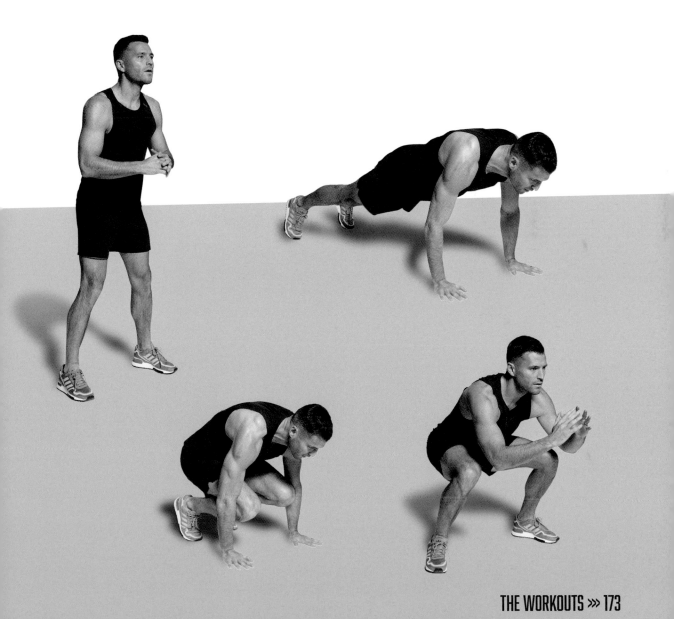

QUICK FEET

Start in a standing position then, on your toes, swap your weight between feet, as fast as you can, performing a tiny sprint on the spot.

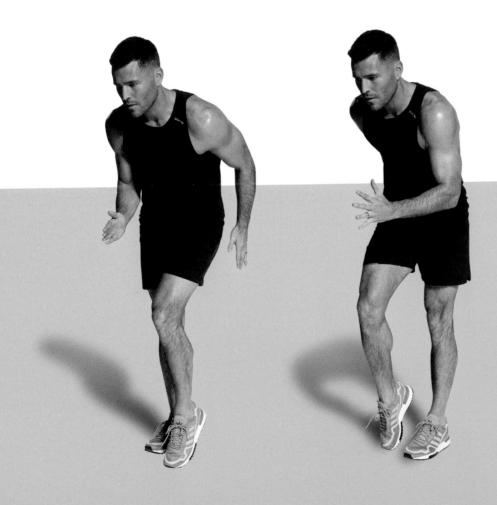

INCHWORM, 3 SQUATS

Start in a standing position, then roll your body down to bring your hands to the floor in front of you, bending your knees. From here, walk your hands forward to bring yourself into a high plank position. Hold for a second then walk both hands back towards your feet and roll your body back up to a standing position. Immediately perform three squats. Repeat.

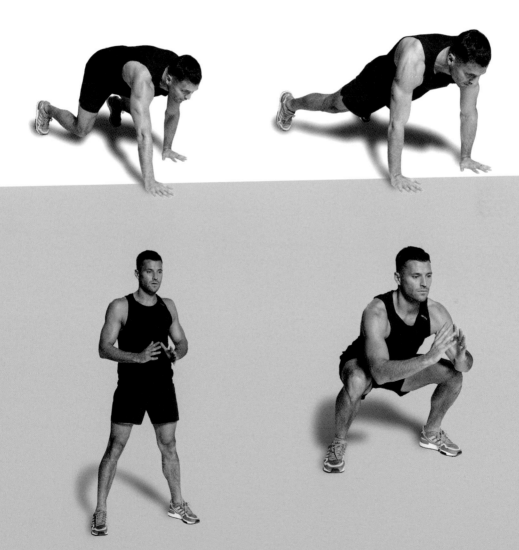

CURTSEY-LUNGE KNEE DRIVES

Start in a standing position, then step your left leg back and to the right of your right leg. Bend both knees to bring yourself down into a curtsey, keeping your chest up. From here, power up and drive the left knee up as quickly as you can up in front of you. Repeat on the opposite side.

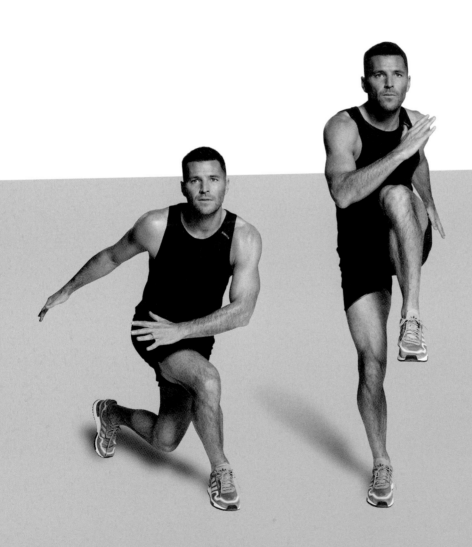

PLANK ROWS

Start in a high plank position, wrists positioned under your shoulders. Lift your right hand and, bending the elbow, squeeze your shoulder blades together and touch your right hip with your hand before returning it back to plank. Repeat on the opposite side.

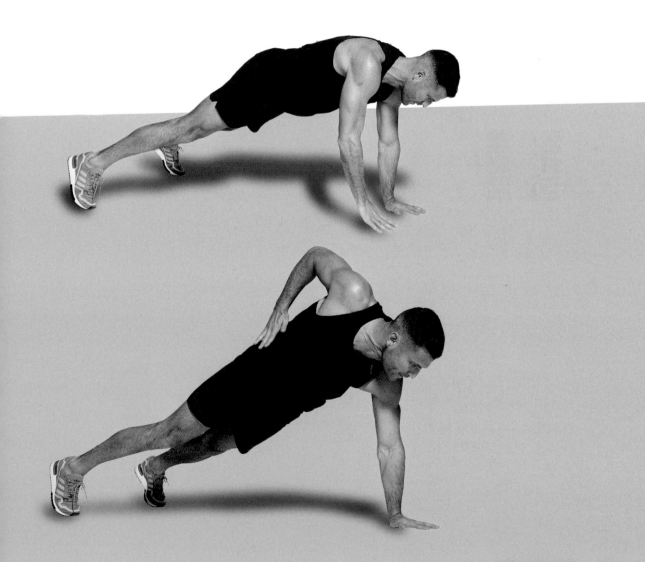

PLANK SIDE WALK

Start in a high plank position, wrists positioned under your shoulders. Lift your left hand and foot and move both a foot to the left and plant them back down. From here, bring the right hand and foot across a foot to the right. Walk the length of your mat/room, then move back in the opposite direction.

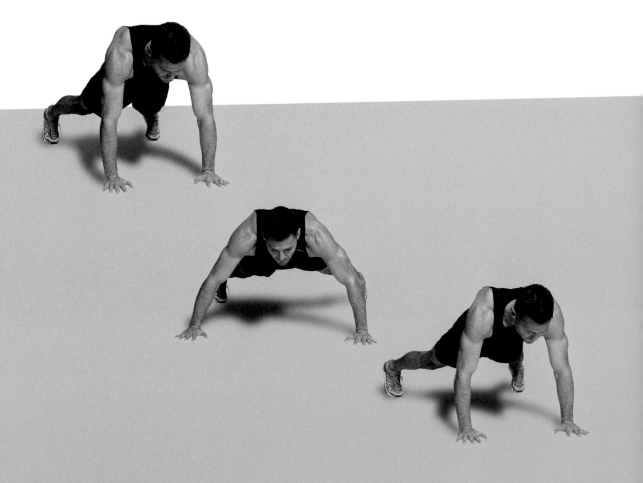

10 HIGH KNEES, 2 DROP SQUATS

Start in a standing position, then drive one knee up to chest height and then the other five times, as fast as you can, to sprint on the spot. Jump both feet wide and bend your knees to bring you into a wide squat, then jump up and bring both feet close together to land. Repeat twice.

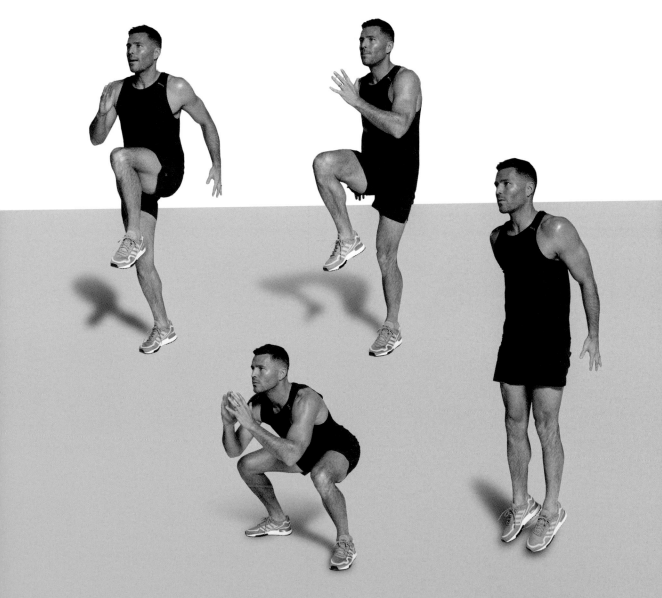

TRICEP DIPS

From a seated position, plant your hands on the floor by your hips and bend your knees. Push into your heels to bring your bum up off the floor and straighten your arms. From here, keep your elbows tight into your body and bend your elbows to bring your body down. When your bum skims the floor, push into your hands and straighten your arms to bring you back to the start. Repeat.

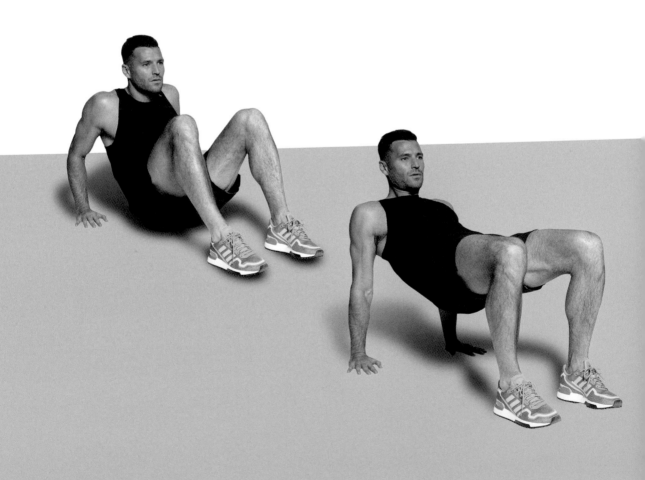

REVERSE-LUNGE KNEE DRIVES

Start in a standing position, then step your left leg back behind you and bend both knees to bring you into a lunge. From here, push off your left foot and quickly drive your right knee up to chest height. Repeat.

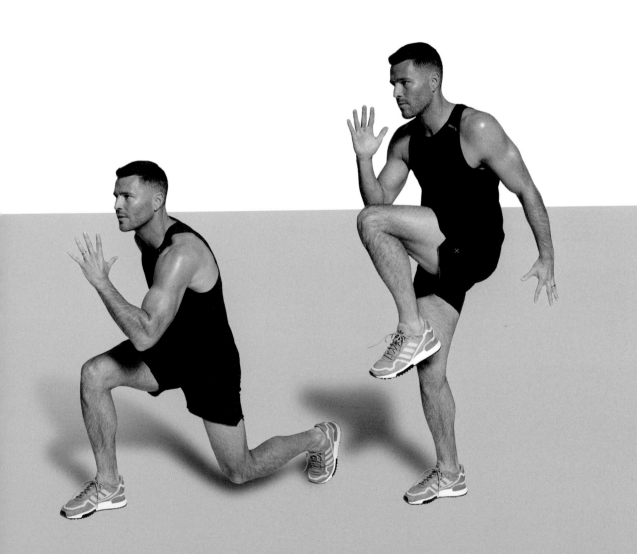

SQUAT PULSES

Start in a standing position with feet wider than hips. From here, sit your bum back and bend your knees to take you into a squat position. Staying low, push into your heels to bring you halfway up, then immediately return to the low squat. Repeat.

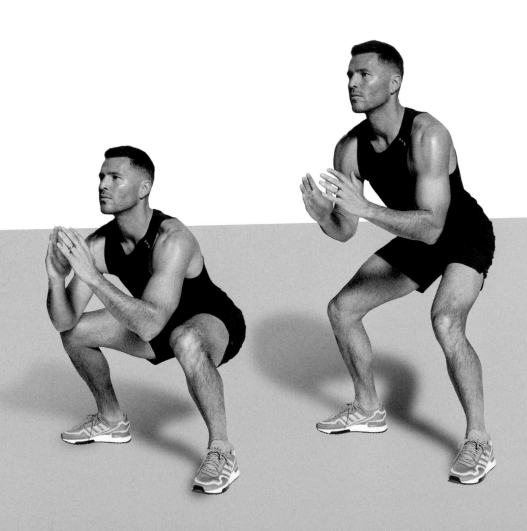

ALTERNATING SIDE LUNGES

Start in a standing position, then step your right leg out laterally to the side, bend your left knee and bring your weight forward over the left knee, keeping your chest up. Push off your left leg to return to standing. Repeat on the other side.

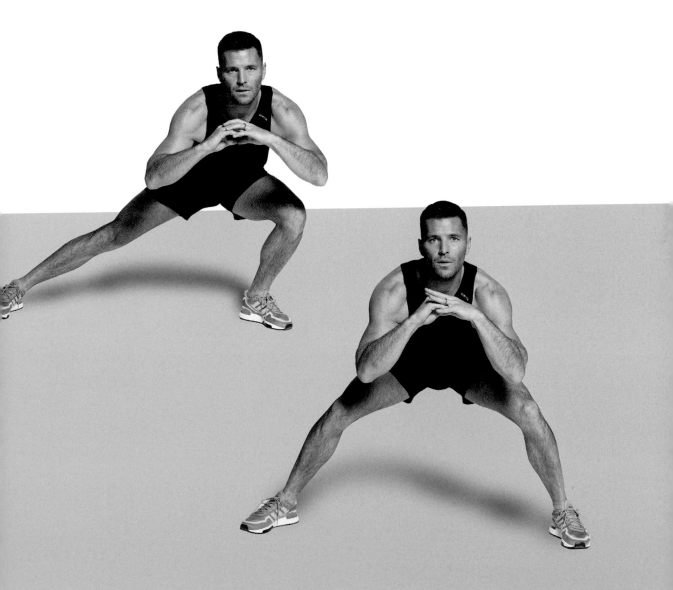

PLANK JACKS

From a low plank position jump both feet out wide, then immediately back into the start position. Keep the core engaged, to keep the body in a straight line. Repeat.

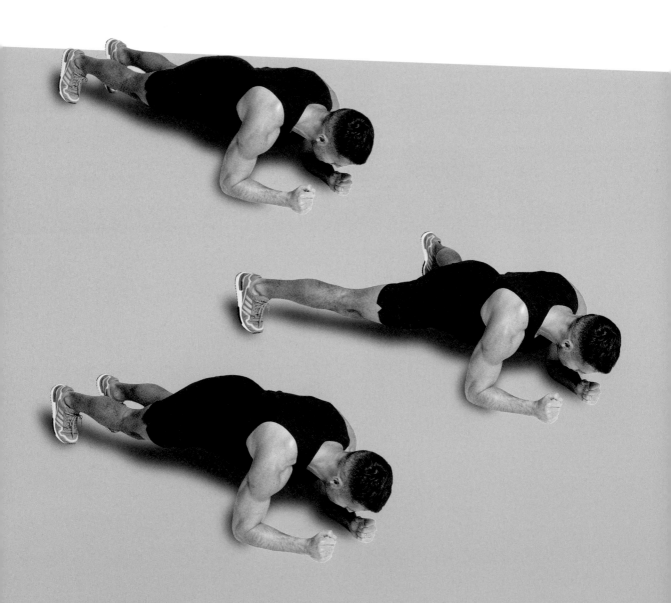

BURPEES

Starting in a standing position, place both hands on the floor and jump both feet back into a high plank position. From here, allow your body to fully drop to the floor. Push into your hands and feet and peel your body off the floor to jump back up to standing. Repeat.

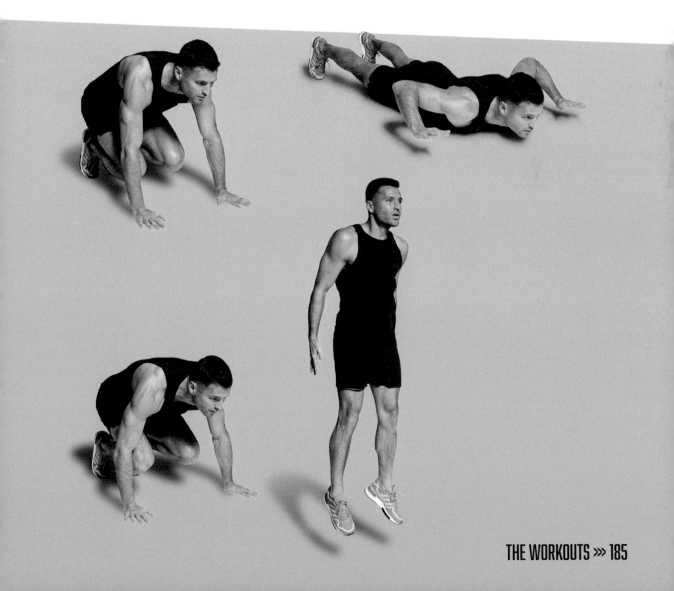

SQUAT HOLD

Start in a standing position with feet wider than hips. From here, sit your bum back and bend your knees to take you into a squat position. Stay low in a static squat for the whole move.

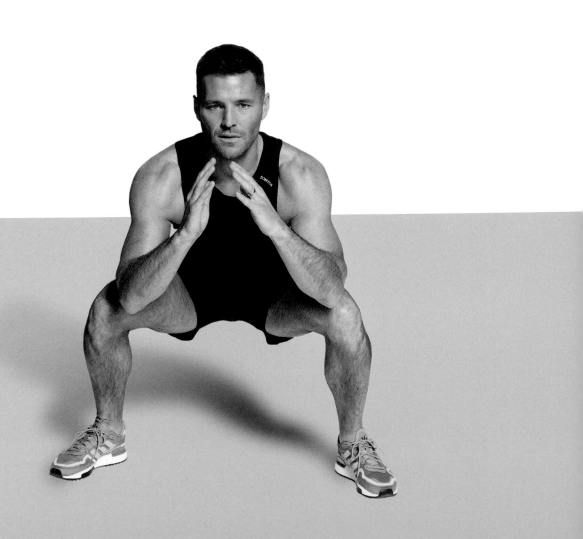

OPEN BODY TWISTS

Start in a high plank position, wrists positioned under your shoulders, then step your right foot up so it is next to your right hand. From here lift your right hand up and to the side until it is directly above your head. Follow your hand with your eyes. Hold for a second at the top before planting your hand back on the floor and stepping your foot back to plank. Repeat, this time on the left side.

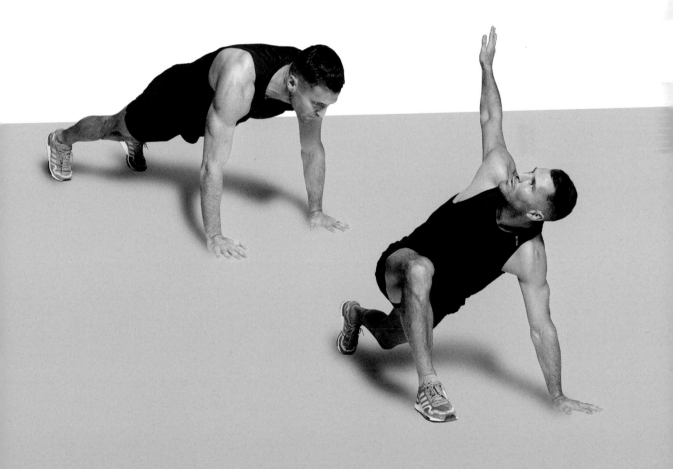

BOXERCIS MOVES

For a lot of these moves you will need to adopt a 'boxer's stance'. How you position yourself will depend on whether you are right- or left-handed. If you are right-handed, stand with the left foot forward and right foot slightly back, with weight in the toes of the back foot. If you are left-handed, swap the legs around. Both hands should be clenched into fists and held up at chin height.

JAB, JAB, CROSS

In a boxer's stance, punch your left hand directly forward with power, chin down. Snap your hand back to your chin while immediately punching your right hand forward. Repeat.

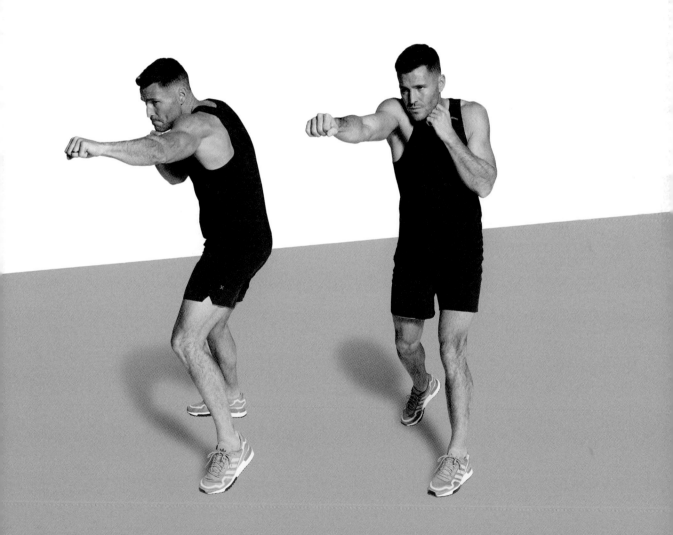

JAB, CROSS, DUCK

Perform one jab cross combination, then bend your knees and drop your bum down and slide it back, then forward and up, as if you're ducking to avoid a punch. Repeat.

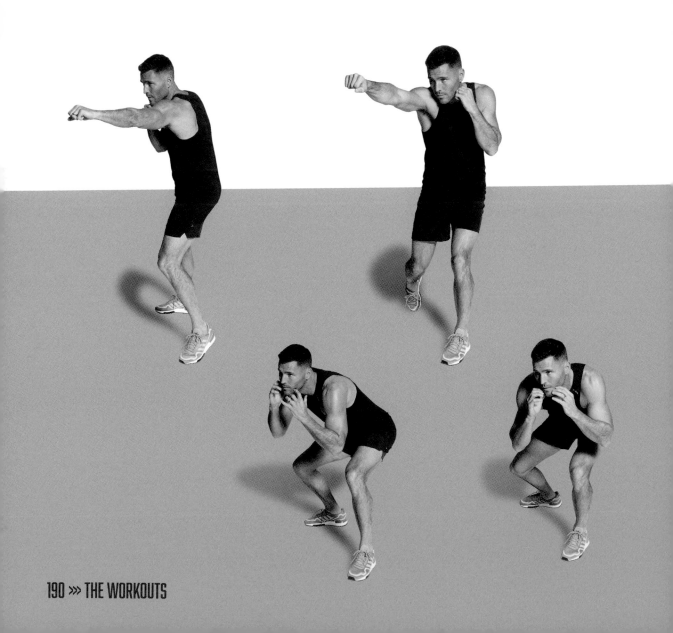

SQUAT-HOLD PUNCH-OUTS

Start in a standing position with feet wider than hips. Sit your bum back and bend your knees to take you into a squat position. Staying low in a static squat, perform quick jab-cross moves.

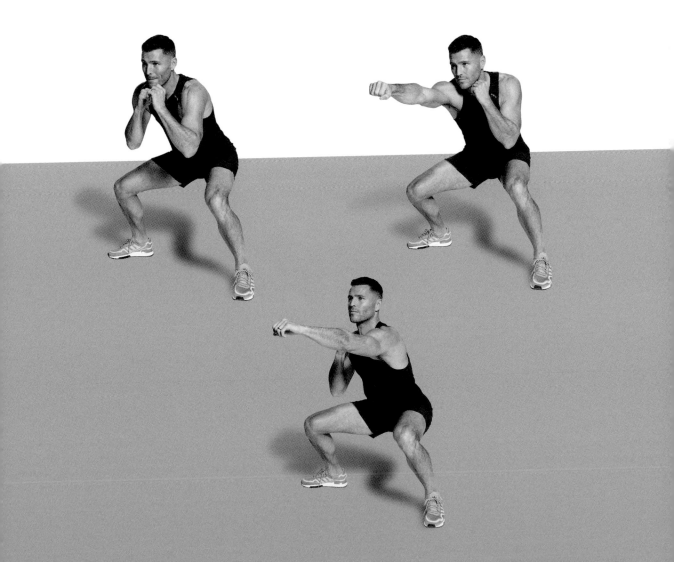

KICK-OUTS

Start in a standing position, then kick your left foot forward in front of you with speed and power. Return to standing, then repeat with the other foot.

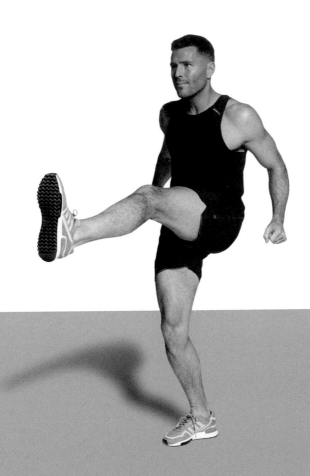

RHYTHM SKIPPING

Start in a standing position and hold an imaginary (or real) skipping rope in your hands. On your toes, quickly shift your weight from side to side as if you are rhythmically skipping.

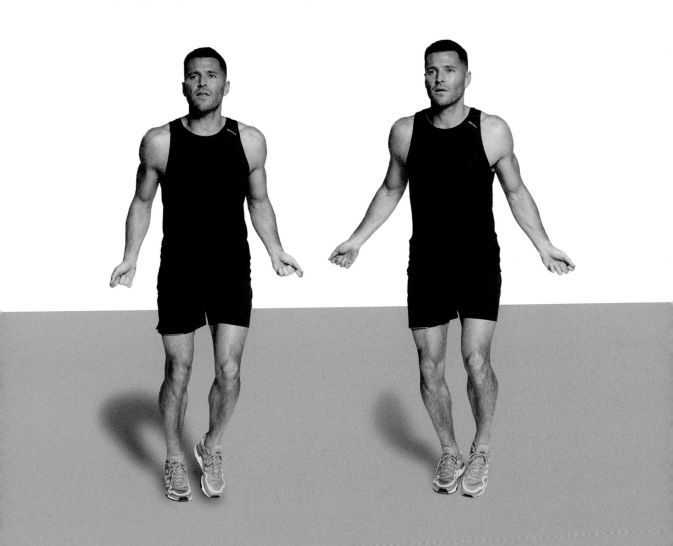

4 JABS, CROSS, SLIDE

Perform two jab-cross combinations then step your front foot forward and slide the back foot behind it. Repeat, but this time stepping backwards.

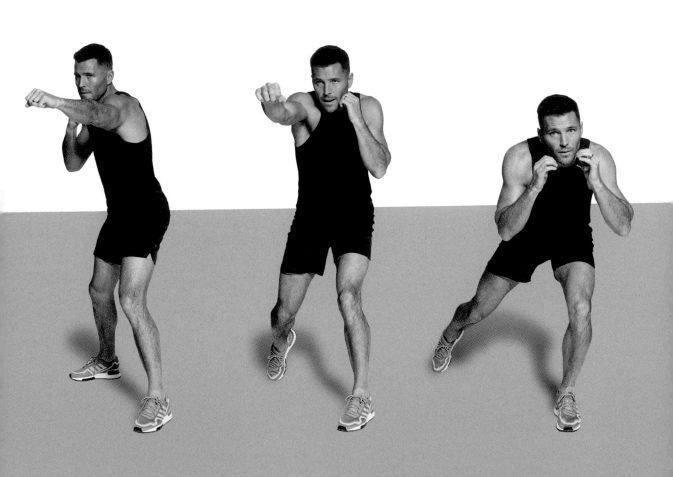

SPRINT-ON-THE-SPOT PUNCH-OUTS

Start in a standing position then sprint on the spot, bringing the knees to a mid-height position (not as high as with high knees) and perform jab-cross punches as fast as you can.

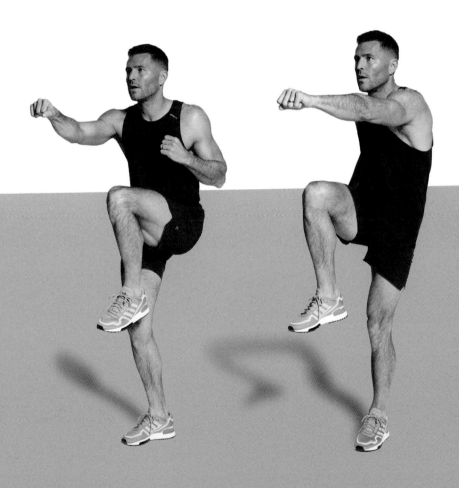

PUNCH JACK SQUATS

Jump down into a squat position, perform two jab-cross combinations, then jump up and bring both feet together to land standing. Repeat.

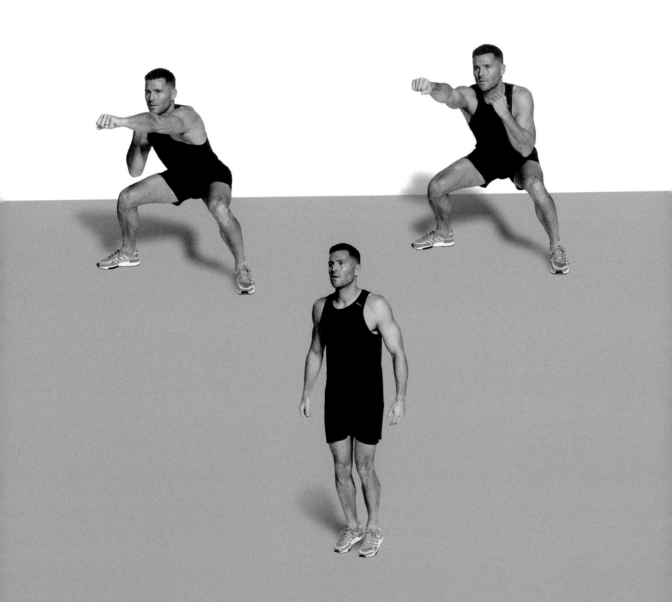

FOOTWORK SWITCH

Start in a boxer's stance then jump up and swap your feet over so the opposite sides are in front and behind. Jump back to the start and repeat.

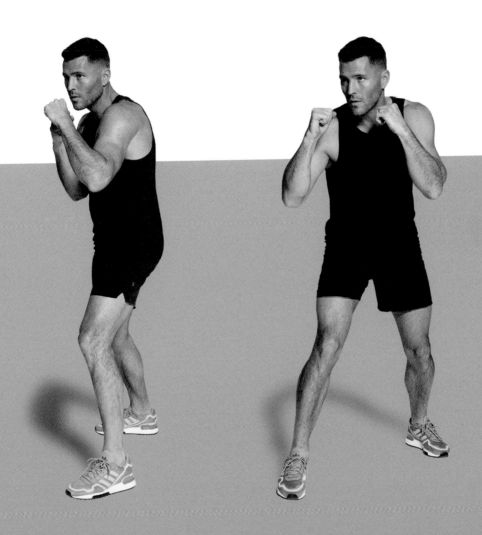

JAB CROSS, ELBOW, ELBOW

Start in a boxer's stance, perform a jab cross, then with your left arm, keep your hand tucked in and drive your left elbow out and round with power. Repeat on the right side.

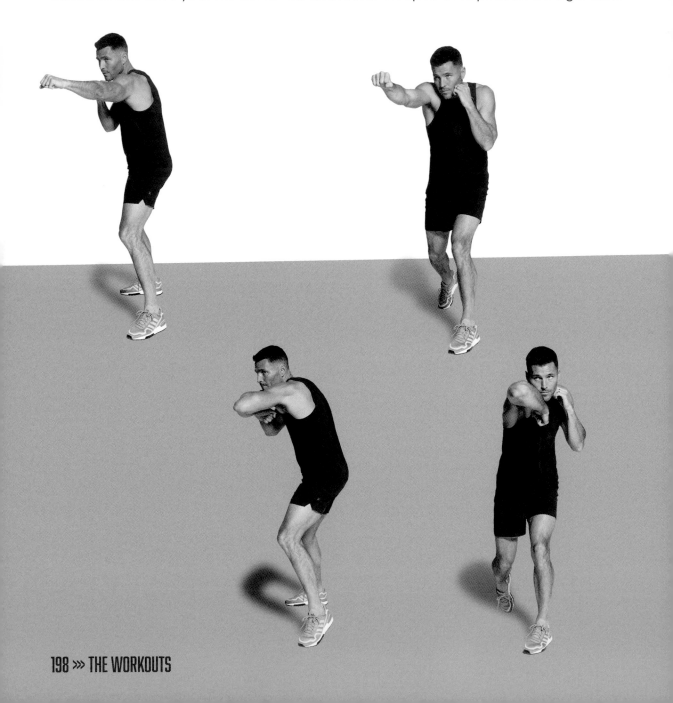

JAB, UPPER CROSS

Start in a boxer's stance and perform a jab punch with your leading arm (left for right-handers and right for left-handers), then bring your opposite hand down and round to bring the fist up from hip height, as if performing a body-shot on your opponent.

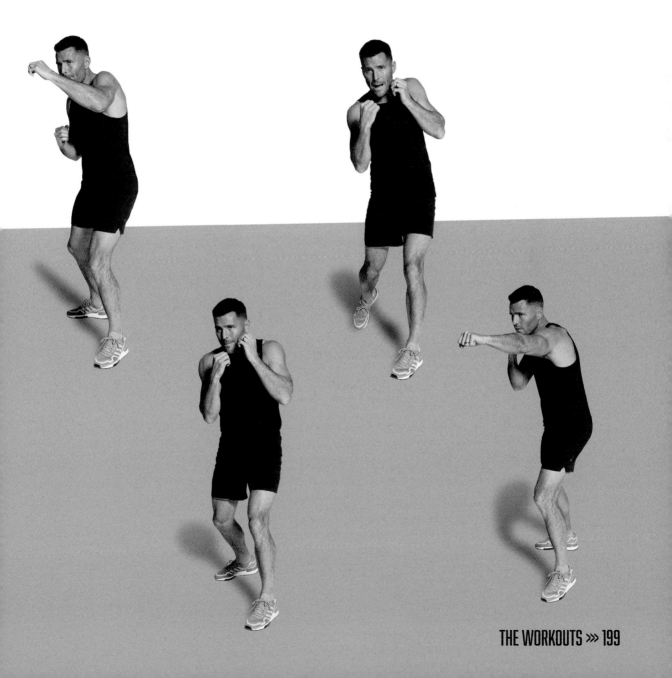

LUNGE JUMP PUNCH-OUTS

Jump up and separate your legs to land in a lunge position, bending both knees. Staying in the lunge, perform a jab cross then jump up and swap the legs over in mid-air to land back in a lunge. Repeat.

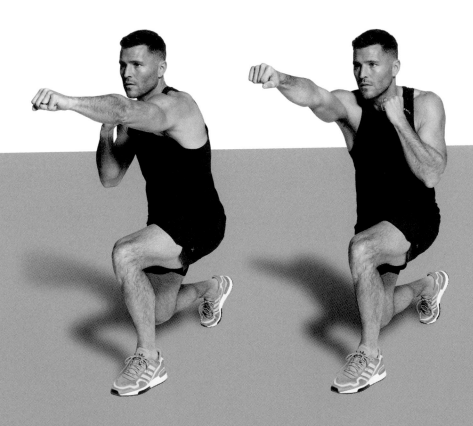

BOXERCISE MOVES
CRUNCH PUNCHES

From a sitting position, plant your heels on the floor and bend your knees. Slowly roll your body down until your back and shoulders are on the floor, and your feet are flat on the floor with knees bent. Use your core strength to peel your body back up to sitting position and, as you do, perform a jab cross at the top of the crunch. Repeat.

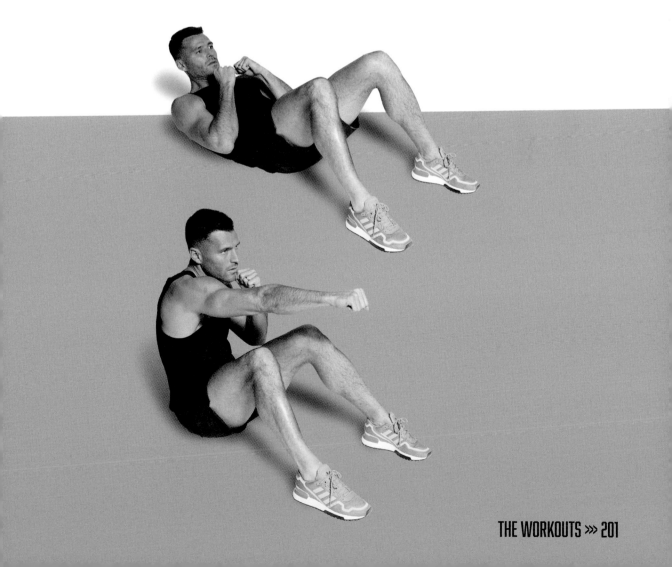

PUNCH-OUT SKATERS

Start in a standing position then, powering off the left foot, jump laterally (sideways) to the right and kick the left foot behind you. From here, keep your balance and perform one jab–cross combination before immediately powering off the right foot and repeat the movement on the opposite side.

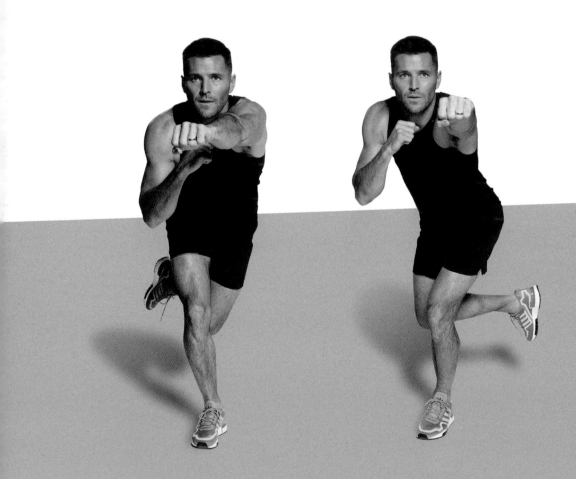

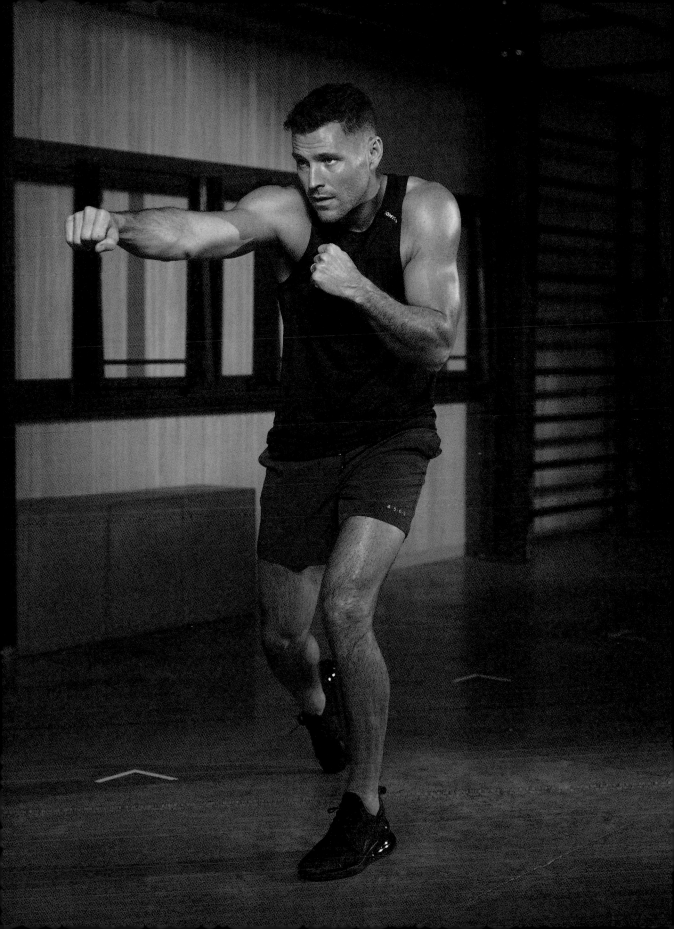

BOXERCISE MOVES
BOXER BURPEES

Start in a standing position and bring both hands to the floor. Jump both feet back into a high plank then jump both feet back to the top, stand up and jump. Once standing, perform one jab-cross combination. Repeat.

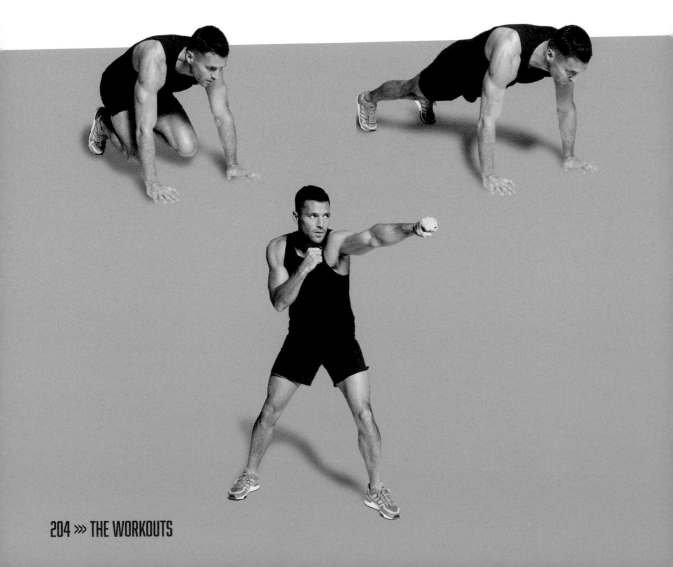

BOXER SHUFFLES

Start in a standing position. Keeping loose at the knees, quickly bring your feet in one at a time, in a bouncing motion. Punch one arm forward in front of you, followed by the other arm. Repeat from the top.

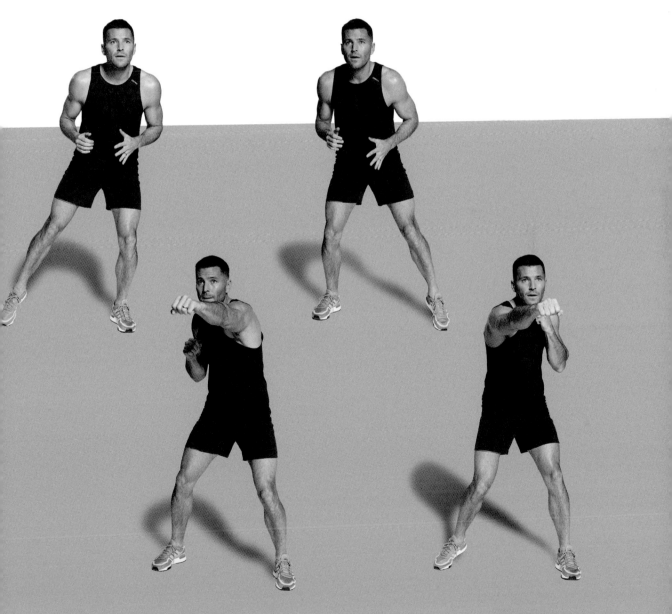

COOL-DOWN AN
STRETCHING

It is really important to stretch regularly when working out, to prevent muscle tightness and aid recovery. Try to incorporate a stretch into your day whenever you train. I've included a few of my favourite stretches here. Perform one, two or all of them, whenever you feel your body could benefit from a stretch.

QUAD STRETCH

Either lying on your side on the floor or standing, bend your left knee and grab hold of your left foot. Keep your knees together and squeeze your heel to your bum to feel a stretch down the front of your leg. Repeat with the other leg.

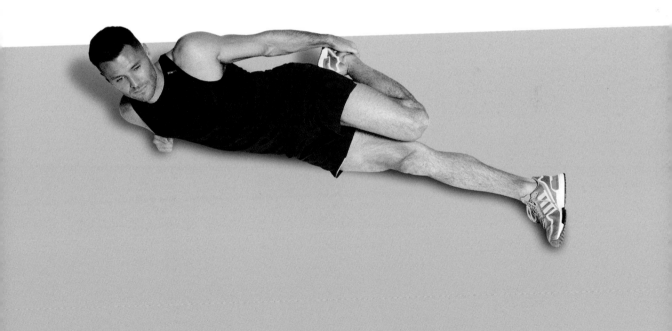

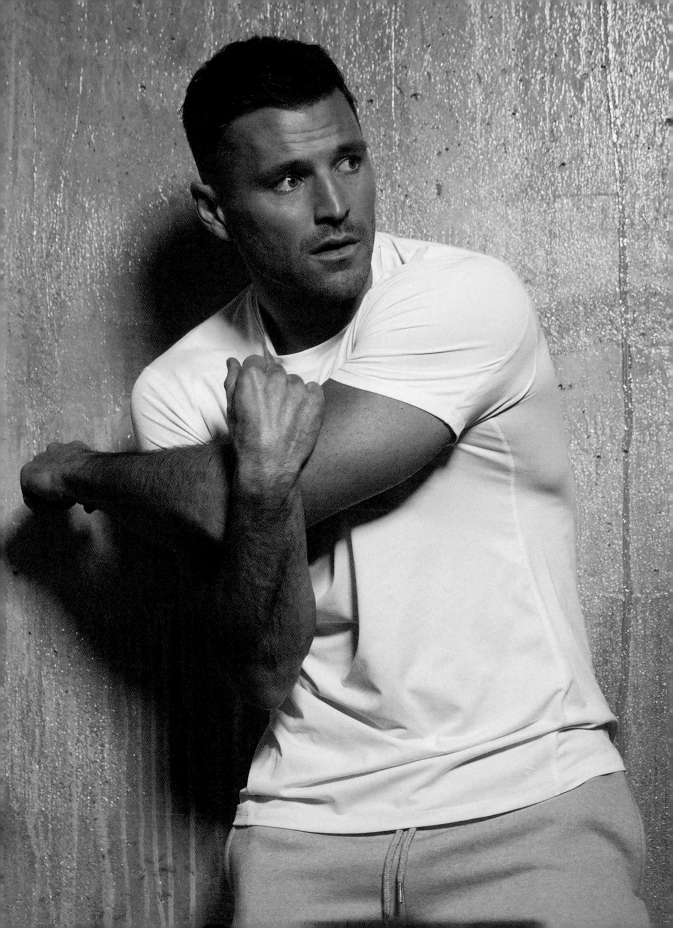

TRICEP STRETCH

Standing or sitting, straighten your left arm across your body then, using your right arm, draw your left arm in tight to your chest to feel a stretch along the bottom of your arm.

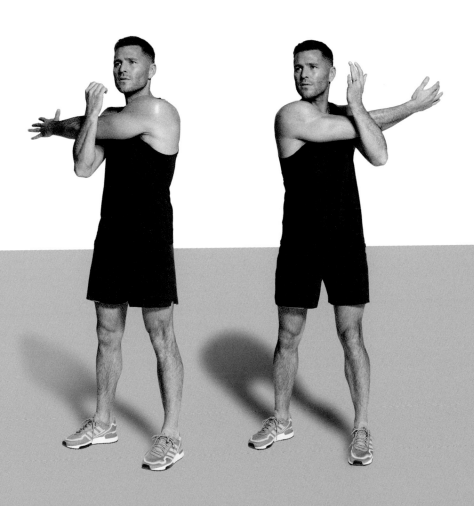

SEATED STRETCH

Sitting on the floor, bring the sole of your right foot to the opposite thigh by bending your right knee. Keeping your chest up, reach for your left shin or toe and hold. Repeat with the other leg.

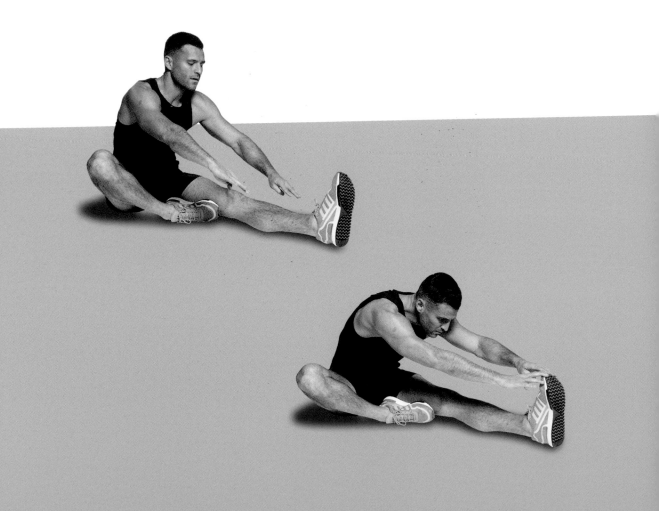

OPEN BODY TWISTS

Start in a high plank position, wrists positioned under your shoulders, then step your right foot up so it is next to your right hand. From here, lift your right hand up and to the side until it is directly above your head. Follow your hand with your eyes and hold for 10–30 seconds. Step back into plank and repeat, this time on the left side.

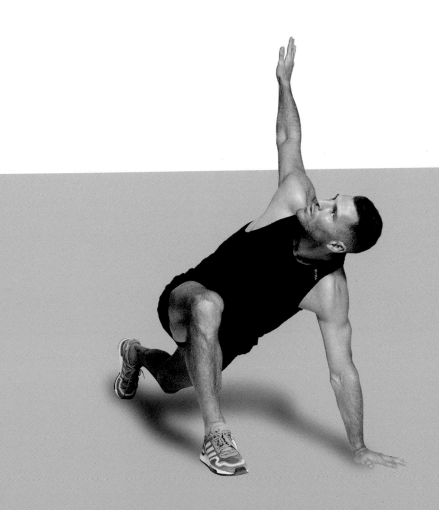

TRAIN WRIGHT SIX-WEEK PLAN

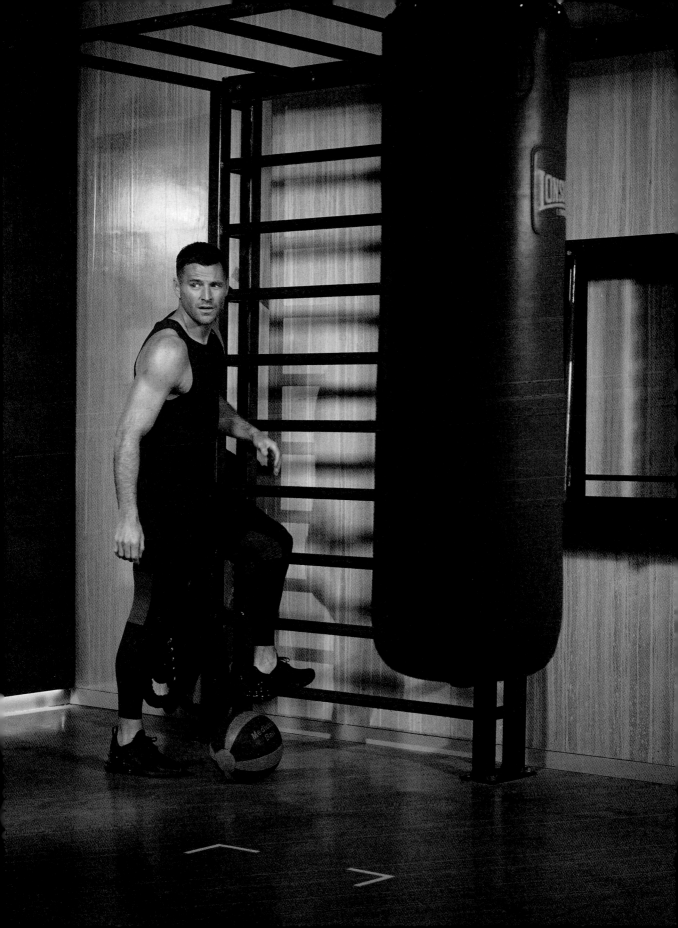

WEEK 1

As excited as you might be to crack on with the fitness side of your journey – and believe me, I can't wait for you to start either – remember, this first week is just the start of your journey.

If you've never worked out like this before, then take this first week in your stride. Pace yourself through the exercises and get to know how your body moves. Make the most of the rest days to recover and take time to notice how much more energy you have and how much better you sleep, to keep you motivated through the week. If you are already a 'gym goer', or have exercised in the past, then use this first week to kickstart a new drive in training. The workouts are all 30 minutes and under, so dig deep and work to your max to get the most out of every session and set the tone for the next six weeks. Enough talk – it's time to get moving.

DAY 1
Pyramid cardio workout

The workout: There are nine exercises to work through in this high-intensity cardio session to kickstart your training plan. The time you work for drops down after each set to max out that heart rate.

The timings: Perform three sets on each exercise.

First set: 45 seconds of work, 15 seconds of rest.

Second set: 35 seconds of work, 15 seconds of rest.

Third set: 25 seconds of work, 30 seconds of rest.

Repeat the whole circuit three times.

The exercises:

1. Shoot-throughs

2. Sprawls

3. Single-arm burpees

3. Inchworms

4. Reverse plank knee-ins

5. Double crossover squats

6. Low-walk twists

7. Running-man lunge jumps

8. Knee-slam burpees

DAY 2

10-Move HIIT workout

The workout: Work to the max with the short sets in this HIIT session. You have just 10 moves to work through, so really push yourself to work as hard as you can for the 25 seconds.

The timings: Perform 25 seconds of work, with 15 seconds of rest and four sets on each exercise before moving on to the next.

The exercises:

1. Full star jumps
2. Knee slams
3. Mountain climbers to plank jacks
4. Press-ups
5. Speed skaters
6. Sprint on the spot
7. Squat jump kicks
8. Knee drives
9. NSEW squat jumps
10. Hops

DAY 3

Three rounds in the ring – boxercise

The workout: Take on three rounds in the ring with this boxing workout. Each round has four exercises to fight your way through for the ultimate cardio session.

The timings: Perform 40 seconds of work, 20 seconds of rest and two sets on each move before moving on to the next. Just one lap of each round.

The exercises:

ROUND ONE

1. Sprint-on-the-spot punch-outs
2. Jab, jab, cross
3. Jab, cross, duck
4. Squat hold punch-outs

ROUND TWO

1. Kick-outs
2. Knee slams
3. Rhythm skipping
4. 4 jabs, cross, slide

ROUND THREE

1. Footwork switch
2. Jab cross, elbow, elbow
3. Jab, upper cross
4. Punch jack squats

DAY 4
Rest day

DAY 5
Bodyweight strength and cardio workout

The workout: The perfect mix of controlled strength moves and high-intensity cardio exercises, this session is designed to build strength and burn fat by using two different timing structures.

The timings: Perform two sets on each of these eight moves before moving on to the next, and two laps of the circuit. The timings for the first and second lap are different:

Lap one: Perform 45 seconds of work and 25 seconds of rest.

Lap two: Perform 25 seconds of work and 15 seconds of rest.

The exercises:

1. Lunge pulses (swap legs for second set)

2. Donkey kicks

3. Frog squats

4. Knees-up punch-outs

5. Squats

6. Cross-body mountain climbers

7. 180-degree squat jumps

8. Press-ups

DAY 6
Your choice of LISS

DAY 7
Rest day

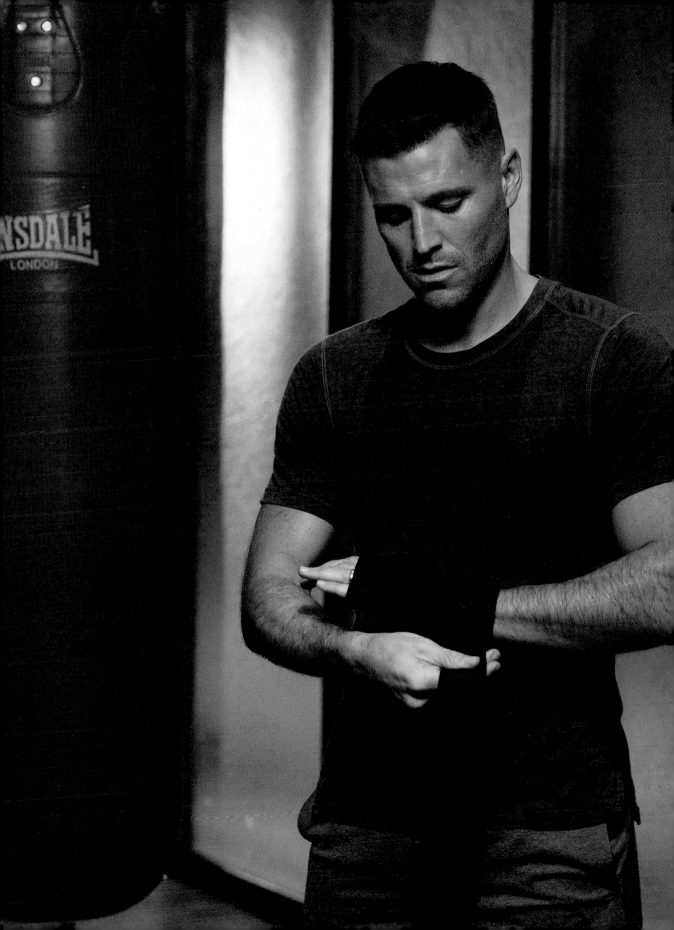

WEEK 2

Here we are already – week two. Your journey is now well underway, which means the hardest part is already done. You've gone further than just buying this book, you've done more than just reading it, you've smashed a whole first week of training. Now your mission is to keep it up. Realise how far you've come already. It might have only been a week but you've moved your body in new ways, which means you'll already have built strength, burnt calories and – no doubt – have been reaping those benefits by feeling amazing. Keep that feeling in mind as you move through week two. An entirely new set of workouts and exercise combinations are coming your way. Stick with it – let's go.

DAY 1
Nine-move HIIT workout

The workout: This is a great workout to kickstart week two. Work through nine high-intensity exercises and four sets on each one. The last set will be tough, but once you've done it, you never come back to that move again. Let's push through every set.

The timings: Perform 35 seconds of work and rest for 15 seconds. Perform four of these sets on each move, then take 30 seconds of rest before moving on to the next. Do just one lap of this circuit.

The exercises:

1. Knee drives
2. Boxer shuffles
3. Reverse plank knee-ins
4. Press up, reach out
5. Cross-body mountain climbers
6. 180-degree squat jumps
7. Plank jacks
8. Toe taps
9. Full star jumps

DAY 2
Two-circuit cardio workout

The workout: Stick to the same timings in this two-circuit cardio workout. Separating out the exercises into two circuits means you get to tick one off halfway through and take a well-deserved rest before taking on circuit two.

The timings: Perform each exercise for 30 seconds and rest for 20 seconds before moving on to the next. Do two laps of the first circuit before moving on to the second. Take a one-minute rest between each circuit.

The exercises:

CIRCUIT ONE

1. Half-burpee squat pulses
2. Quick feet
3. Inchworm, 3 squats
4. Curtsey-lunge knee drives
5. Press up, reach out

CIRCUIT TWO

1. Mountain climbers
2. Plank side walk
3. 10 high knees, 2 drop squats
4. Squats
5. Single-leg donkey kicks (swap legs for second set)

DAY 3
Bodyweight strength workout

The workout: This full-body session slows things down a bit and uses your bodyweight to burn calories and build strength. Make sure you remember to switch legs between sets so each side is worked equally.

The timings: Perform two sets on each exercise, working for 40 seconds and resting for 20 seconds. When you reach the end of lap one, take a one-minute rest before you return to the start and repeat for a second time.

The exercises:

1. Forward bear crawl
2. Tricep dips
3. Alternating side lunges
4. Press up, reach out
5. Reverse-lunge knee drives
6. Low plank hold
7. Squat pulses

DAY 4
Rest day

DAY 5
Four, three, three-formation boxercise

The workout: Use your boxing skills to smash out the calories in this session. Four laps of three rounds means you are kept on your toes in this workout.

The timings: Perform one set on each move, working for 45 seconds and resting for 15 seconds. Work through the three rounds four times in total, taking a one-minute rest between each full lap.

The exercises:

ROUND ONE
1. Punch jack squats

2. Footwork switch

3. Jab cross, elbow, elbow

ROUND TWO
1. Jab, upper cross

2. Lunge jump punch-outs

3. Crunch punches

ROUND THREE
1. Punch-out skaters

2. Punch jack squats

3. Boxer burpees

DAY 6
LISS day

DAY 7
Rest day

WEEK 3

Okay, week three is here, which means you've now smashed two whole weeks of exercise.

I'm hoping that, by now, you are getting used to the formats of the workouts, enjoying the variation, and are learning when it best suits you to fit them into your day. These things are all just as important as doing the workouts. You are learning how to fit exercise into your week, feeling the benefits of regular movement and, hopefully, noticing that it really doesn't take hours to do it. Keep that momentum up and don't be tempted to skip a day – only YOU can keep going, no one else can do it for you, so find that determination I know you have.

Also, keep in mind that once this week is through, you're halfway through the plan!

DAY 1
Nine-move HIIT workout

The workout: Simple but effective, this workout is made up of nine exercises and four sets on each one. After you've done the exercise for four sets, put it in the cupboard, it's done, you never do it again during this workout.

The timings: Perform 35 seconds of work and rest for 15 seconds. Perform four sets on each move then take 30 seconds of rest before moving on to the next. Do just one lap of this circuit.

The exercises:

1. Toe taps

2. Inchworms

3. 10 high knees, 2 drop squats

4. Forward bear crawl

5. Running-man lunge jumps

6. Knees-up punch-outs

7. Crunch punches

8. Low-walk twists

9. Knee drives

DAY 2
Cardio and core blast workout

The workout: Work to your max with three circuits of high-intensity moves and a one-minute plank at the end of each one. This session gets your heart rate sky high, burning fat and giving you that big hit of endorphins to take away with you. The cheeky one-minute plank at the end of each circuit builds some serious core strength.

Timings: Perform 40 seconds of work and 20 seconds of rest and two sets on each exercise before moving on to the next. At the end of each circuit hold a one-minute plank, then take 30 seconds of rest before starting the next circuit.

The exercises:

CIRCUIT ONE

1. Burpees

2. Reverse plank knee-ins

3. Donkey kicks

4. Sprawls

ONE-MINUTE PLANK

CIRCUIT TWO

1. Curtsey-lunge knee drives

2. Rhythm skipping

3. Jump jack step-outs

4. Plank jacks

ONE-MINUTE PLANK

CIRCUIT THREE

1. Speed skaters

2. Squat jump kicks

3. Hops

4. Quick feet

ONE-MINUTE PLANK

DAY 3
Rest day

DAY 4
Half-and-half workout

The workout: Work through one circuit of bodyweight strength and one circuit of HIIT cardio for the perfect mix. This session uses every muscle in the body to get a decent sweat and burn all in one.

The timings: Perform 35 seconds of work and 20 seconds of rest on each exercise. Perform two laps of each circuit before moving on to the next.

The exercises:

CIRCUIT ONE – BODYWEIGHT STRENGTH

1. Squat hold
2. Shoot-throughs
3. Squats
4. Plank side walk
5. Low-walk twists
6. Press up, reach out
7. Frog squats

CIRCUIT TWO – HIIT CARDIO

1. Half burpees
2. Sprint on the spot
3. Full star jumps
4. Mountain climbers to plank jacks
5. Squat to 4 high knees
6. Jump jack step-outs
7. Boxer shuffles

DAY 5
Rest day

DAY 6
Knockout boxing HIIT workout

The workout: You are back in the ring for this boxing workout. Today the sets are long, so pace yourself to make it through all the way to the end of each one. Use the longer rest to catch your breath and prepare for the next move.

The timings: Perform one minute of work on each exercise with 30 seconds of rest before moving on to the next. Do three laps of the circuit in total.

The exercises:

1. Knee slams
2. Jab, jab, cross
3. 4 jabs, cross, slide
4. Footwork switch
5. Lunge jump punch-out
6. Hops
7. Punch jack squats
8. Boxer burpees
9. Squat jump kicks

DAY 7
LISS day

WEEK 4

You absolute legend, you are halfway through already and you are absolutely smashing it.

Before you rush on to see what the next workout is – and how many burpees I'm going to get you to do – just take a little moment to slap yourself on the back for keeping it up. If you are anything like me, I'm sure there were days where you had to have a lot of conversations with yourself, debating whether or not you were going to do it. But you did, and it's important to remember that and carry that with you, remembering how good it felt when you actually did it, into week four. Keep up the healthy eating and positive mindset alongside these workouts and you'll be another week into that healthier lifestyle change. Okay... now you can work out!

DAY 1
Whole-body HIIT workout

The workout: It's the beginning of week four and what better way to kickstart it than with this full-body HIIT circuit. Just nine moves to work through today – get it done.

The timings: Perform four sets on each exercise. For the first two sets, perform 20 seconds of work, 10 seconds of rest. For the second two sets perform 45 seconds of work, 25 seconds of rest.

The exercises:

1. NSEW squat jumps

2. Running-man lunge jumps

3. Cross-body mountain climbers

4. Squat knee to elbow

5. Knee-slam burpees

6. Tricep dips

7. Inchworm, 3 squats

8. Broad jump, jump back

9. Sprint on the spot

DAY 2
Rest day

DAY 3
Six-move boxercise pyramid workout

The workout: Strap yourself in for rounds of boxing skills. Starting with the longest time per set, as the rounds move on, the time you work for decreases and so should the effort you put in. Finish by smashing out a two-minute plank.

The timings: Perform four laps of these six exercises, one set on each. Take a 30-second rest between each lap.

First lap: 1 minute work, 30 seconds rest.

Second lap: 45 seconds of work, 25 seconds of rest.

Third lap: 30 seconds of work, 15 seconds of rest.

Fourth lap: 20 seconds of work, 10 seconds of rest. At the end of all four rounds, hold a two-minute plank to finish.

The exercises:

1. Jab, jab, cross

2. Quick feet

3. Jab, cross, duck

4. Kick-outs

5. Jab cross, elbow, elbow

6. Punch jack squats

TWO-MINUTE PLANK TO FINISH

DAY 4
Rest day

DAY 5
Bodyweight strength and cardio workout

The workout: Work through three circuits in today's session. Each circuit has three specially selected bodyweight strength moves to help you build strength and tone, and ends with a one-minute cardio sprint on the spot.

The timings: Perform 45 seconds of work, 25 seconds of rest on each of the three exercises and two sets on each exercise before moving on to the next. After sprinting on the spot for 1 minute, take 1 minute of rest before moving on to the next circuit.

The exercises:

CIRCUIT ONE

1. Alternating side lunges

2. Squat hold

3. Plank rows

ONE-MINUTE SPRINT ON THE SPOT

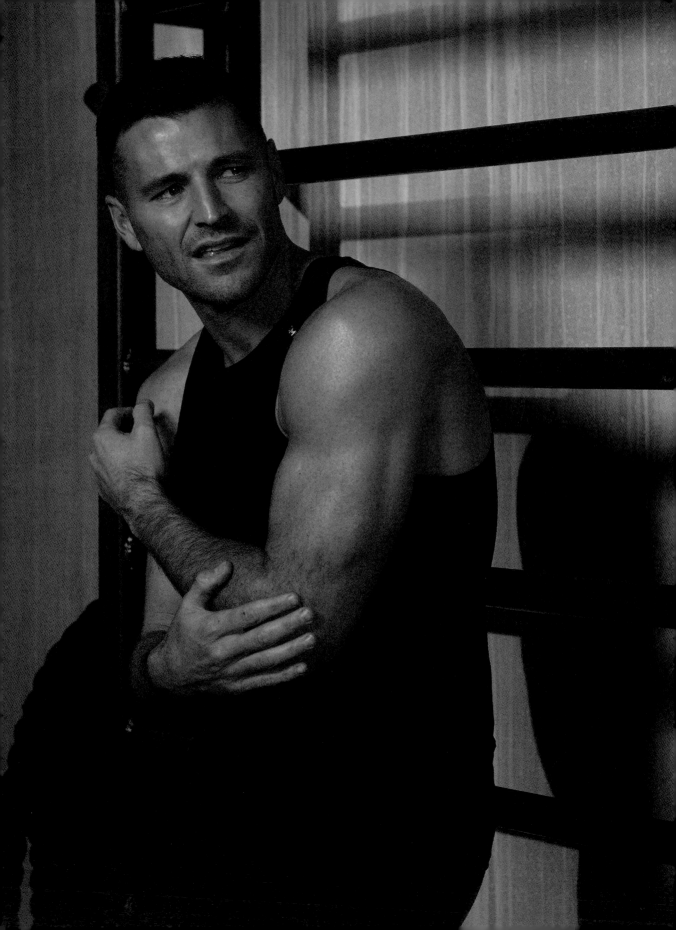

CIRCUIT TWO

1. Frog squats

2. Forward bear crawl

3. Lunge pulses

ONE-MINUTE SPRINT ON THE SPOT

CIRCUIT THREE

1. Open body twists

2. Shoot-throughs

3. Squats

ONE-MINUTE SPRINT ON THE SPOT

DAY 6
LISS day

DAY 7
Three sets HIIT workout

The workout: Finish off the week strong with this beast of a HIIT workout. Loads of moves to keep things changing and the timings stay the same throughout. Max out those 35-second sets and you'll be reaping the benefits in just 30 minutes.

The timings: Perform three sets on each exercise before moving on to the next. For each set, do 35 seconds of work, with 15 seconds of rest.

The exercises:

1. Press up, reach out

2. Full star jumps

3. Mountain climbers

4. Squat pulses

5. Knees-up punch-outs

6. Single-arm burpees

7. Squat pop twists

8. Forward bear crawl

9. Curtsey-lunge knee drives

10. Speed skaters

11. 10 high knees, 2 drop squats

12. Alternating side lunges

WEEK 5

Week five guys, and we're starting the week with a rest day. Resting between workouts is so important, not only to give the body time to recover, but also to help push you through the workout days. It's as simple as this: if you know you've got a rest day coming up, you'll be way more likely to work harder and really push yourself as hard as you can to achieve more, because you know you'll get that well-deserved rest the following day. You know the benefits by now, you know how good you feel after the exercise and for the rest of the day, so there is nothing else to say but… let's crack on.

DAY 1
Rest day

DAY 2
Three rounds in the ring – boxercise workout

The workout: Take on three rounds in the ring with this boxing workout. Each round has four exercises so let's dig deep and push hard on every single one.
The timings: Perform 40 seconds of work, 20 seconds of rest; two sets on each move. Perform one lap of each round.

The exercises:

ROUND ONE

1. Punch jack squats

2. Boxer burpees

3. Rhythm skipping

4. Kick-outs

ROUND TWO

1. Half burpees

2. Jab, jab, cross

3. Crunch punches

4. Footwork switch

ROUND THREE

1. Footwork switch

2. Jab cross, elbow, elbow

3. Jab, upper cross

4. Punch jack squats

DAY 3
Pyramid cardio workout

The workout: There are nine exercises to work through in this cardio session and the time you work for drops down after each set to max out that heart rate. Pace yourself on the longer sets and sprint as hard as you can on those 25-second sets towards the finish line.

The timings: Perform three sets on each exercise.

First set: 45 seconds of work, 15 seconds of rest.

Second set: 35 seconds of work, 15 seconds of rest.

Third set: 25 seconds of work, 30 seconds of rest.

Repeat the whole circuit three times.

The exercises:

1. Running-man lunge jumps

2. Knee slams

3. Squat jump kicks

4. Hops

5. Broad jump, jump back

6. Half burpees

7. Sprawls

8. Single-leg donkey kicks

9. Inchworm, 3 squats

DAY 4
LISS day

DAY 5
Two-lap HIIT circuit workout

The workout: You have eight high-intensity moves to get through – twice – in this high-intensity cardio session. By the time you finish the second lap you'll be absolutely buzzin'. Let's go.

The timings: Perform two sets on each of these eight moves before moving on to the next, and two laps of the circuit. The timings for the first and second lap are different:

Lap one: Perform 45 seconds of work and 25 seconds of rest.

Lap two: Perform 25 seconds of work and 15 seconds of rest.

The exercises:

1. Knees-up punch-outs

2. Jump jack step-outs

3. Squat knee to elbow

4. Toe taps

5. Broad jump, jump back

6. Boxer shuffles

7. Half burpees

8. Open body twists

DAY 5
Rest

DAY 7
Two-lap bodyweight strength workout

The workout: You can't get bored in this workout as you work through 13 different bodyweight exercises. Designed to get every muscle in the body fired up, you will also work on building your core strength with that cheeky little one-minute plank at the end of each lap.

The timings: Perform one set on each exercise, working for 45 seconds and taking 25 seconds of rest. At the end of the first lap, perform a one-minute plank and take a one-minute rest before returning to the top to take on lap two.

The exercises:

1. Press-ups

2. Squat knee to elbow

3. Open body twists

4. Shoot-throughs

5. Low-walk twists

6. Press up, reach out

7. Curtsey-lunge knee drives

8. Plank side walk

9. Squats

10. Tricep dips

11. Lunge pulses

12. Reverse-lunge knee drives

13. Squat pulses

ONE-MINUTE LOW PLANK HOLD

WEEK 6

You've made it. The final week in the plan. I don't need to tell you to dig deep and carry on, because if you've come this far, you've already done that yourself. Week six isn't the start of the last week of exercise, or the last time you are going to cook up a healthy, balanced meal; week six is simply the end of the first chapter in your fitter, healthier, happier life. While this six-week plan was set out to challenge you, it was also designed to help you make the changes you've been wanting to make in your life for a while. Five weeks in, you've proven to yourself that you CAN move more, you CAN make healthier meal choices and you CAN reap all the benefits that come with it. Once this week is complete, I know you aren't going to just close this book and go back to a life without regular exercise, because I know how amazing you are feeling right now and how much you'll want to keep that feeling for years to come. This week, let's enjoy every workout, push harder to burn those extra few calories and finish off the last week of the beginning of your journey so we can crack on with every single healthy week that is going to follow after it.

DAY 1
Tabata HIIT circuit workout

The workout: It's short sets, short rests and high reward in this cardio session. Because the sets are only 20 seconds long, you need to dig deep and work with maximum effort on every single one to get the most you can out of this sweaty circuit.

The timings: Perform five sets on each move, working for 20 seconds with 10 seconds rest.
Do just one lap of the circuit.

The exercises:

1. Crunch punches
2. Knee slams
3. NSEW squat jumps
4. Hops
5. Knees-up punch-outs
6. Half burpees
7. Shoot-throughs
8. Sprawls
9. Running-man lunge jumps
10. Single-leg donkey kicks
11. Quick feet
12. Plank rows

DAY 2
Rest

DAY 3
Ultimate boxercise circuit workout

The workout: Go for the knockout with this boxing sesh. By working through 15 different moves you are constantly changing things up to keep your body challenged and your mind sharp.

The timings: Perform three sets on each move and one lap of the circuit. For the first two sets, perform 20 seconds of work with 10 seconds of rest, then for the third set, perform 40 seconds of work with 20 seconds of rest before moving on to the next move.

The exercises:

1. Jab, jab, cross
2. Jab, cross, duck
3. Squat hold punch-outs
4. Kick-outs
5. Rhythm skipping
6. 4 jabs, cross, slide
7. Sprint-on-the-spot punch-outs
8. Punch jack squats
9. Footwork switch
10. Jab cross, elbow, elbow
11. Jab, upper cross
12. Lunge jump punch-outs
13. Crunch punches
14. Punch-out skaters
15. Boxer burpees

DAY 4
Reverse pyramid cardio workout

The workout: These nine exercises promise to leave every muscle in the body feeling fired up and your mind ready to face the day. The length of the sets increase as you go through, so pace yourself at the start then sprint to the finish.
The timings: Perform three sets on each exercise before moving on to the next.
First set: 25 seconds of work, 30 seconds of rest.
Second set: 35 seconds of work, 15 seconds of rest.
Third set: 45 seconds of work, 5 seconds of rest.
Repeat the whole circuit three times.

The exercises:

1. Mountain climbers

2. Speed skaters

3. Knee drives

4. NSEW squat jumps

5. Sprint on the spot

6. Burpees

7. Frog squats

8. Half-burpee squat pulses

9. Plank side walk

DAY 5
Rest

DAY 6
Three-circuit HIIT workout

The workout: Work through three different circuits of exercises in this high-intensity session. Each circuit contains four exercises that promise to get you working to your max, building strength and burning fat.
The timings: Perform 40 seconds of work and 20 seconds of rest on each exercise and one set on each one. Once you reach the end of the circuit, return to the start to complete a second lap before moving on to the next circuit.

The exercises:

CIRCUIT ONE

1. Footwork switch

2. Burpees

3. Mountain climbers to plank jacks

4. Squat knee to elbow

CIRCUIT TWO

1. Full star jumps

2. Knee slams

3. Press-ups

4. Toe taps

CIRCUIT THREE

1. Broad jump, jump back

2. Inchworms

3. Single-leg donkey kicks

4. Plank rows

9. Burpees

10. Inchworm, 3 squats

11. Mountain climbers

12. Jump jack step-outs

13. Double crossover squats

14. Quick feet

15. Sprawls

DAY 7
Ultimate HIIT finisher

The workout: This is it, the last workout in your six-week plan, and we're going to make sure we bring maximum energy to show how far we've progressed. Working through 15 exercises means we are constantly changing the movements, keeping our bodies – and minds – working hard. Come on, let's finish on a high.

The timings: Perform two sets on each of these exercises, working for 40 seconds and resting for 20 seconds. Perform just one lap of the circuit.

The exercises:

1. Speed skaters

2. Sprint on the spot

3. Reverse plank knee-ins

4. Running-man lunge jumps

5. Knee drives

6. Squat pulses

7. Plank jacks

8. Half burpees

A FINAL WORD – KEEPING THE WRIGHT BALANCE

I'm so proud of you for getting this far. You've not only completed the six-week plan, but instead of closing the book and going back to where you were when you opened it, you've turned the page to see what happens next. This is exactly what this book is all about – not just giving you a plan to follow, but guiding you through a change of lifestyle that, by now, will have you feeling so amazing you can't wait for the next chapter. And the good news is, that next chapter is for the taking. You are now armed with all the tools you need to keep up the good work. You know you can make time for regular exercise – and how amazing you feel when you do. You know how to make changes to your diet to eat well, without going hungry. And you know how to balance out good sleep and healthy habits with a good social life and all those slightly less healthy things that come with it.

I've loved sharing my story with you and I hope it has helped to show you that no one starts life knowing how to balance out a healthy lifestyle, but that we can all achieve it with the right mindset.

TESTIMONIALS

I haven't spoken much about how it feels seeing the transformation pictures of people who have taken on my workout plans, but every time I see images like this it's just the best feeling in the world. It only feels right that, when I share the journeys of these incredible people, I throw mine in there too. Everyone starts somewhere and taking a picture when you begin a journey is such a powerful thing to look back on. Mine is a month's journey. I'm not saying that in the first picture that I'm completely out of shape, but for me, I was feeling far from my best. After making changes for a week I felt so much happier, more motivated and healthier. That's what I see in these pictures. The difference between how people hold themselves in their before pictures compared to their after shots shows everything. The change in confidence is clear to see.